A Special Kind of Doctor

A Special Kind of Doctor
A History of the College of Community Health Sciences

By PATRICIA J. WEST
with WILMER J. COGGINS, M.D.

College of Community Health Sciences of The University of Alabama
Tuscaloosa

Copyright © 2004
College of Community Health Sciences of The University of Alabama
All rights reserved
Manufactured in the United States of America

Distributed by The University of Alabama Press
Tuscaloosa, Alabama 35487-0380

Typeface: ACaslon

∞
The paper on which this book is printed meets the minimum requirements of
American National Standard for Information Science–Permanence of Paper for
Printed Library Materials, ANSI Z39.48-1984.

Library of Congress Cataloging-in-Publication Data

West, Patricia J. (Patricia Jean), 1963–
    A special kind of doctor : a history of the College of Community Health Sciences /
by Patricia J. West with Wilmer J. Coggins.
        p. cm.
    Includes bibliographical references and index.
    ISBN 0-8173-1429-6 (cloth : alk. paper)
    1. University of Alabama. College of Community Health Sciences—History.
2. Family medicine—Study and teaching—Alabama—History. I. Coggins, Wilmer J.
II. University of Alabama. College of Community Health Sciences. III. Title.
    R746.A2 W47 2004
    610′.71′176184—dc22

                                                                    2004000604

Contents

Photographs follow page 93

Preface

In the spring of 1970, David Mathews, Wayne Finley, John Burnum, Dick Rutland, and others committed themselves and The University of Alabama to an intensive experiment unique in the history of academic medicine. Their purposes were three-fold: 1) to address the need for physicians in rural Alabama; 2) to counter the trend toward technology-driven, expensive, and impersonal patient care; and 3) to expand the definition of health and of health professions education to include the community as essential and central to such a model. The result was the College of Community Health Sciences (CCHS). To give life to their vision, three key components of CCHS from the start were a Family Practice Residency; community-based education for medical students, residents, and other health professions students; and community-responsive research and outreach. At every level, the approach was to be interdisciplinary.

The early team was soon to expand to include John Packard, Bobby Moore, Bob Pieroni, David Hefelfinger, and a "Kentucky Mafia" emigrating with Willard from the new University of Kentucky College of Medicine, including Bill Winternitz, Roland Ficken, Doug Scutchfield, Russ Anderson, and Bob Gloor. So as Americans walked on the moon, as the war in Vietnam became a raging controversy, and as students demonstrated and rioted on campuses across the nation, Mathews, Willard, and company forged a new kind of college, with a new kind of mission, with a new kind of name.

As we approached the thirtieth anniversary of the founding of CCHS, it was apparent to me that for most of the CCHS family of alumni, students, residents, staff, and even faculty, our knowledge of the CCHS story was limited—mostly limited to tales of the rivalries between CCHS and the larger UA medical campus in Birmingham. While knowing the truth about that part of the story was necessary, a history restricted to that perspective alone was sure to be lacking in many ways. CCHS Dean Emeritus Wilmer Coggins has given generously of his time and skill to head a superb effort of volunteers and staff to produce this story.

It is a story not just about the struggles—academic, financial, political, or personal—but about the reasons for those struggles: the purposes born of the efforts of our founders, and the results we can claim over those thirty years. It is important to know the truth about it all, because knowing it frees us for today's work. Surely it is so that he who ignores the lessons of history is condemned to repeat them. Beyond that, parts of the story have national implications, both in medical education and in the realm of public policy, and are as relevant today as then.

However, in sifting the facts and plotting the vectors of the past thirty years, an even more substantial reason for studying the history of CCHS emerges. It is that in doing so we can establish relationships with the minds and hearts that brought the experiment to life. We have the limited opportunity to get to know the people who did it, because many of the founders and early leaders are still with us. Not only are they able, but willing, to recall, to reflect, and—many of them—to spend considerable time in writing and refining the story. For them, as well as for students, residents, patients, and communities of people in Alabama and indeed across the nation—we can be grateful. They have contributed to a rich and fulfilling journey.

The journey begun amidst exploding azaleas and dogwoods, confronting exploding technology, health care costs, and emerging dissatisfactions about the American system of health care, has continued. The routes have been both predictable and surprising. The reasons for the founding of CCHS are if anything more pertinent today than they were thirty years ago: rural communities have even more complex medical, economic, and social distress; American health care is even more technology-driven, expensive, and impersonal; and the role of "community" in health care and in other essential relationships and decision making faces an uncertain future.

The people of our state and nation are crying out for something different, something to clarify and balance the whole confusing system. If we are going to participate in the discussion, we still need the vision of thirty years ago, refined and adapted for today. We still need physicians and others educated and trained with an extra dimension, an additional set of tools in their black bags. We still need a special kind of doctor.

William A. Curry, M.D., F.A.C.P.
Dean, CCHS

Acknowledgments

This book would not have been possible without the insightfulness of Dean William A. Curry, who recognized the need to record a history of the college as the program reached its thirtieth year in 2002. He asked former dean Roland Ficken to bring a small group together to establish the guidelines for the book and to suggest its general tenor. This group included Drs. John Burnum, Richard Rutland, Riley Lumpkin, William Winternitz, Will Coggins, and Mrs. Lisa Rains Russell. Over a period of three years, this group worked to make this book a reality.

Of this group, Mrs. Russell deserves special recognition. Throughout the entire process she remained dedicated to the project, meeting with the editor and writer each week, helping with research, writing, editing the manuscript, and identifying others who mined the archival ores in the university libraries in Birmingham and Tuscaloosa. We are especially grateful for her loyalty throughout this process.

Mrs. Nelle Williams, interim director of the Health Sciences Library, and her assistant, Mrs. Sharon Glenn, have provided valuable assistance in finding sometimes obscure, even unreferred material from libraries throughout the United States. The book would not exist without their help.

Dr. Samuel E. Gaskins wrote a virtually complete history of the family practice residency, where he has served as director of the residency program since 1980, except for a brief interlude. Dr. James Leeper, former chair of the community medicine program, has done likewise, giving us a history of that department's activities from the beginning to the present. We are grateful for their contributions.

Some thirty faculty, staff, and administrators in Birmingham and on the University of Alabama campus in Tuscaloosa have been interviewed, or have provided responses by letter to our questions. They will be identified as they are quoted in the text.

Special thanks are due to Ms. Barbara S. Lord, who provided staff support to the initial planning group, not knowing that she would be expected to staff the efforts of the production team for the ensuing two and a half years. She has provided order to our efforts, and has done so graciously.

We have been fortunate to have been given working space in the dean's administrative offices where Mrs. Vicki Johnson, director of Advancement, and Mrs. Linda Wright, Ms. Pat Murphy, Mrs. Carol Boshell and their student assistants have cheerfully responded to our requests for material support, and assistance in copying and communication. They have provided a pleasant and supportive atmosphere in which to work.

Mrs. Linda Jackson, editor of the college newsletter "On Rounds," has been an invaluable resource for dates and data from that source and others.

Ms. Nickole L. Moore, with her long service to the CCHS surgery department, provided a comprehensive view of that department's activities over the years.

Ms. Mary Kay Hannah graciously made the resources of the medical student affairs office available to us.

Two University of Alabama graduate students contributed to the book: Mr. Edward Black in the history department conducted archival research for the project in its early stages. Ms. Brook Darnell in the library school conducted research for us for many months as we attempted to fill in the holes in our story.

Mr. Thomas Land of the University of Alabama archives and records management group also provided useful information, as did Mr. Tim Pennycuff of the University of Alabama at Birmingham's archives.

Ms. Laura Green and Mr. Timothy Martin of DCH Regional Medical Center helped identify and provide the photograph of the hospital used in this book.

Many other individuals assisted us by providing materials, often retrieved from their personal files, that helped tremendously: in particular Dr. James Pittman, Dr. Riley Lumpkin, Ms. Judy Hodges, Professor Richard Thigpen, and Dr. John Packard.

This manuscript was improved by several individuals who agreed to read or review parts of it, including Dr. Charles Lydeard, Ms. Anne R.

Gibbons, Ms. Patricia Norton, Dr. Roland Ficken, and Dr. Richard O. Rutland.

U.S. Senator Richard Shelby provided useful background about the early development of the college, for which we are grateful.

We also appreciate the financial support provided by the Lister Hill Society, headed by Mr. Tommy Hester. This book would not have been possible without its support.

Introduction

To many, the term "family doctor" conjures up an image of a kindly older man, caring, knowledgeable, dependable. Perhaps he has a small office, a small staff, and a steady stream of patients that have known him for twenty years or more. In all probability he has been a part of many major family events, including the arrival of the new baby, that broken bone, perhaps even the death of an elderly family member. He was someone the family trusted absolutely to provide solid medical advice, comforting words, and reassurance that everything would be all right.

But what if you lived in a town that had no such person? No family doctor to whom you could turn to when the baby got sick, when hay fever season hit, or when someone you loved contracted that first virus of the season. Such was the case in many of the nation's small towns and rural communities during the fifties and sixties and beyond. Medical help might be fifty miles or more away, perhaps in the form of a distant emergency room or the office of a physician whom you had never met. "Family doctor" in this case was an abstraction, a physician who cared for *other* families, in *other* cities or towns.

The University of Alabama's College of Community Health Sciences was established in 1972 to help address this problem in Alabama, where the doctor shortage was severe. Here, the nation's serious paucity of physicians was heightened due to the predominantly rural population of the state. While substantial increases in physicians in the state were occurring in the five largest counties, the number of doctors in the other sixty-two counties was declining. Although the population of the state was growing, largely in the urban centers, the output of new doctors had not kept pace.

But the distribution of doctors was not the only reason for the doctor shortage. Many of the new doctors being trained were choosing the more prestigious specialties or subspecialties of medicine, and were choosing to practice them in the more urban areas of the state. Family medicine, so widely practiced before World War II, had rapidly been replaced by specialized areas of expertise. By 1970 fewer than 15 percent of medical school graduates in the United States chose to enter careers in family or general practice.

Something needed to be done. In response the Alabama Legislature turned to the University of Alabama and its range of resources to address the health demands of the state. A study of the situation soon helped to determine that the answer did not lie entirely in the production of more physicians. What was needed was a special kind of doctor trained in the area of family medicine, general practitioners who would choose to practice in the state's underserved small towns and rural communities and who were equipped to treat the myriad of basic medical problems found in those areas.

Family medicine became a new specialty of primary care in 1969. Trained to provide comprehensive personal health care, the "new" type of physician was to act as the first point of contact for the patient, to evaluate his or her total health needs and assume responsibility for those needs in the context of the community and family.[1] Dr. G. Gayle Stephens, former dean of the School of Primary Medical Care at the University of Alabama School of Medicine in Huntsville summarized the distinctions that characterized family physicians.

> Family physicians know their patients, know their patients' families, know their practices, and know themselves. Their role in the health care process permits them to know things in a special way denied to all those who do not fulfill this role. The true role of family medicine lies in the formalization and transmission of this knowledge.[2]

CCHS was established to fulfill the need for more family doctors for rural Alabama but also to educate an "undifferentiated" physician—one who chose to attend the community-based campus but would go on to the traditional specialties. The college is a unit of both the University of Alabama and the University of Alabama School of Medicine (UASOM) in Birmingham, an academic health center of national rank established in 1945. Yet in spite of close ties between the two institutions, the Tuscaloosa program was not an outgrowth of the medical school in Birmingham. Indeed, these two institutions, with their distinctive goals and missions, were often at odds during the developmental years of the medical education program in Tuscaloosa. Absorbed in medical research and highly technical approaches to treatment, and concerned about the meager education dollars available in the impoverished state, administrators and faculty at UASOM were skeptical about this program designed to train family doctors and to develop different models for health care delivery.

Today, in spite of this uneasy beginning, CCHS is helping to meet the state's needs by providing physicians with the expertise to provide accessible, up-to-date, and compassionate medical care in two basic ways: the education of medical students and the training of medical school graduates in the specialty of family medicine. The undergraduate medical education program in Tuscaloosa provides the clinical years of medical education for UASOM medical students who choose to explore opportunities in primary health care: family medicine, general internal medicine or pediatrics. Medical students who choose to join CCHS first complete two years of basic sciences, known as the preclinical phase of medical school, in Birmingham before embarking on the clinical two years in Tuscaloosa. The curriculum for third- and fourth-year medical students consists largely of bedside instruction, a clinical experience that allows a small group of students, usually fewer than four, to be taught by a faculty physician in the appropriate specialty, as the group "makes rounds" on their hospital patients each day. CCHS students are trained in patient care at both DCH Regional Medical Hospital and the Capstone Medical Center, the university's outpatient clinic. CCHS students also have a preceptorship in Family and Community Medicine through a rural medicine clerkship (Appendix C).

The second important component of the CCHS program is a well-established family practice residency, a three-year training program for newly graduated physicians who wish to specialize in family practice. The specialty allows physicians to gain the experience they need to perform as family physicians, who would have the first contact with patients. The first resident arrived on the UA campus in 1974 and now thirty-six of these doctors are in training in Tuscaloosa each year (Appendix D).

A major aspect of our community-based medical education program is the use of private practitioners as teachers for the medical students and residents. Many of the surgical and medical specialists in Tuscaloosa provide experience for both medical students, principally in their senior year, and for residents during the second and third years of training.

This book covers three distinct topics, the first being an overview of medical education in the state, with an emphasis on the public medical schools that served as the predecessors to CCHS. This material provides perspective on the development of the college and why its development was necessary in Alabama. This preliminary material will also serve to acclimate readers who may be unfamiliar with the history of medical education. The second section deals with the motivation for creating such a program. The final chapters outline the history of the college, from its uncertain beginning to the flowering of this program that has provided its unique contribution to the health care of the people of Alabama.

This book is a history of an institution: as such it recounts the development of facilities, programs, and outcomes. But in larger measure the book serves as a history of the dedicated and enthusiastic people who helped to make a special kind of doctor for the people of Alabama.

A Special Kind of Doctor

I

Medical Education in Alabama

The Early Years

The University of Alabama School of Medicine (UASOM) in Birmingham can trace its origins to the heart of the city of Mobile. Here in 1859 the Alabama Medical College was established, a small institution started by a local physician who recognized the need for more doctors for the state. Although a handful of other medical schools were established in Alabama in the middle of the nineteenth century, only this institution would have a lasting impact on the training of physicians in Alabama.

U.S. medical education differed greatly from the format that we know today. In the mid-1800s, medical school consisted only of attendance at a course of lectures, usually lasting six weeks. The same lectures were repeated once each year, and students were encouraged to attend a second time. Typically, this didactic teaching took place after a year of apprenticeship with a practicing physician who was willing to be observed and to have the service of an assistant in his practice. This experience, in addition to the equivalent of a high school diploma, was all that was required for admission to medical school. With such low entrance requirements and courses that were perfunctory and brief, the process was quite informal: it took relatively little work to become a physician.[3] Few schools required any type of exam for graduation and licensing by states was not yet a practice. Becoming a medical doctor, therefore, consisted primarily of "claiming to be one."[4]

Those who were dissatisfied with this cursory approach to medical education could pursue more vigorous postgraduate training in Europe. France and Germany, in particular, were considered the "mecca" of foreign medical study, teaching pathology, laboratory methods, physical diagnosis, and the statistical method of clinical research.[5] Those who studied there had a decided advantage.

The Start of Medical Education in Alabama

Formal medical education did not begin in Alabama until 1859. At that time the noted surgeon Dr. Josiah Clark Nott of Mobile convinced the people of that city to support the establishment of a medical school. Nott was a well-respected surgeon, scientist, and ethnologist who had received wide attention for his 'scientific' views on the inherent inferiority of blacks to whites.[6] Nott also established himself as a pioneer in American medicine as early as 1848. Many years before the germ theory was proven Nott had pointed out his belief that yellow fever was probably transmitted by mosquitoes, not by vapors from swamps or other environmental factors, which was the standard belief of the day. He reached this conclusion after careful observation of the pattern of outbreaks of yellow fever in Mobile and elsewhere.

Nott had long tried to convince the legislature to support such a venture, arguing the merits of educating the state's physicians within its borders, rather than losing them to other states. Nott himself had been educated at the medical school of the University of Pennsylvania, one of the oldest and best-known educational institutions in America at the time. When the state refused to support the medical school, Nott was able to convince some of his wealthy and influential friends to fund such a school without assistance from the state. Using rented quarters, Nott started his remarkable school, equipped with the latest in teaching aids and models, which he had purchased during an extended trip to Europe using funds donated by the citizens of Mobile. When Nott and his faculty of seven full-time professors opened the doors of the medical college in 1859, one hundred and eleven students were enrolled.

The school was deemed an immediate success, and shortly thereafter, the state agreed to participate in this venture and appropriated $50,000 for a building. The school, with its superior museum of anatomical models and new facility, was a source of pride for Nott, who referred to it as his "own creation and hobby." In 1860 the college became the Medical Department of the University of Alabama but had its own board of trustees. Nott's success in getting both governmental and private support for the new school preceded by half a century Abraham Flexner's attack on proprietary medical schools, in which faculty depended on student tuition fees for their salaries.

The medical college represented the state's first attempt at medical education, but it was not to last. The outbreak of the Civil War in 1861 forced the closure of the school as both students and faculty (including Nott) left to join the war effort.

When the war ended, the building that had housed the medical college was taken over by the Freedmen's Bureau, which used the facility as a primary school for newly freed blacks. Nott, unable to convince the government to return the building to its original purpose, moved his family to New York where he established a private medical practice.

Some physicians in Mobile persisted in trying to open the medical school again, and they were successful by the fall of 1868. However, Alabama was destitute after the war, and the legislature was only able to provide the school with funding in the amount of $5,000 per year.[7] In spite of this, the school slowly grew again as more students were admitted and faculty were added. Likewise the curriculum was improved, but the struggling school was unable to keep pace with developments that were revolutionizing medical education in the United States. Elsewhere, lectures and recitations were rapidly being replaced by laboratory and clinical work, a form of teaching that required greater financial resources than were available to the administrators of the school.

Another major effort to provide medical education in the state took place in growing Jefferson County in 1894, when nine local physicians opened the Birmingham Medical College. Entrance requirements were the same as in Mobile: an apprenticeship with an established physician and a high school diploma or the equivalent. In spite of the limitations of the school, it was successful and filled an important niche in North Alabama.[8] Over the years the institution grew: a new building was constructed to house the school in 1902 and the faculty was expanded. In 1903 the school contracted with the Hillman Hospital, a ninety-eight-bed hospital built with funding by industrialist Thomas T. Hillman, then president of the Tennessee Coal, Iron and Railroad Company. The new arrangement helped provide an important clinical function for the school, especially since the faculty physicians were given control of the hospital.

Medical Education Reformed

Like so many of the medical schools operating during this time, the Birmingham and Mobile schools were operating in the proprietary model, that is, they were run for profit. Like many others, they were owned and operated by the faculty, who collected their salaries from the fees and tuition of the students, although Nott's intention had been to separate tuition from support for the teachers.

All in all, these institutions were autonomous and self-sufficient, but often woefully underfunded. Furthermore, stiff competition between schools at the national level made a "farce" out of medical education.[9] Not surprisingly, many disagreed with this profit-oriented approach to medical education, believing that the interests of business naturally conflicted with those of education. Yet, public funds for medical schools as such were not widely available at this time, even though many other educational institutions were supported by local and/or state funds. The school in Mobile was something of an exception as the legislature did provide $5,000 to help pay faculty salaries and to support a tuition grant to one indigent student from each county in the state.

But this was soon to change. Concern over the numerous deficiencies in medical education became a nationwide concern, and by the 1860s and 1870s, change was on the horizon. One of the primary issues was the fact that medical practice was not keeping pace with medical knowledge.[10] Great strides had been made in medicine in the previous fifty years: the germ theory of infectious disease had been verified, leading to a decline in infections and death; anesthesia had been introduced, making surgery more effective; and advances had been made in the diagnosis and treatment of disease, especially infectious diseases.

However, such landmarks were not always reflected in the classroom. Many schools of the day lacked laboratories, which had been demonstrated to be necessary for the study of microbiology, histology, pathology, and physiology. Furthermore, to the disadvantage of many medical students, many instructors were older physicians who had not kept pace with the developments in the field or, alternatively, had trained at institutions of lesser quality.

Slowly, teaching techniques evolved. Learning became more hands-on as courses of study emphasized clinical and laboratory work and minimized didactic teaching. Although the new approach and the associated techniques were held up as the ideal, these changes were costly to implement. Needed were well-equipped laboratories, additional faculty, and control over a teaching hospital, which few schools could afford, especially those that relied on meager student fees.[11] It was not until university medical schools came to be more common in the early 1900s that such changes could be fully realized.

Major improvements were made at a few key schools during this time, changes that would break ground and ultimately lay the foundation for many dramatic developments in the decades to come. One of the first universities to embark on a major upgrade to the medical curriculum was Harvard University, where the medical school was made to be an integral part of the university, the course of instruction was lengthened, and teaching methodology was improved.

The next event of significance was the opening of Johns Hopkins Medical School in 1893, which set high admission standards, kept classes small, and had a hand-picked and talented faculty, a generous endowment, and a true university spirit. Furthermore, it emphasized clinical teaching that essentially transformed the hospital ward into a medical classroom. Thus, Johns Hopkins represented a radical departure from other institutions and soon became the recognized ideal, heralding the beginning of medical education as we know it today.

Such changes, as sweeping as they were, were clearly not enough, since only a handful of the nation's medical schools had made such upgrades. Throughout the continent, almost two hundred others staggered along in their old ways. Realizing this, attempts to regulate the nation's system of medical education began in 1904. At that time, both the American Medical Association (AMA) and the newly formed Association of American Medical Colleges (AAMC) devised a system for evaluating and rating medical schools. This would stimulate some change in medical education, causing many medical schools to close and others to increase funding. The changes, however positive, were small compared to what lay ahead.

Flexner and the Changing Face of American Medical Education

The most profound changes in medical education took place in 1910 as a result of the publication of a report commissioned by the New York–based Carnegie Foundation for the Advancement of Teaching, *Medical Education in the United States and Canada*. At the time, the foundation had undertaken a critical study of all the medical schools in the United States and Canada in response to national concern about the quality of medical education. The study of the medical schools was conducted for the good of the public, "in accordance with the finest conceptions of public service."[12] Thus, for the first time, medical education across the country had been thoroughly investigated with the intent of upgrading a clearly inadequate system.

The resulting report was largely the work of Abraham Flexner, who joined the Carnegie Foundation in 1908, and was charged with conducting the study. Although trained and previously employed as an educator, with little knowledge of what medical education entailed, Flexner quickly familiarized himself with the issues in North America and set out to visit and review the 155 schools in operation at the time. After two years of fieldwork and writing, Flexner issued his highly critical report, which came to be known as the Flexner report.

The report, among other things, was notable for its scathing and colorful details on the conditions of the existing medical schools. Comments such as "dirty and disorderly beyond description," "an embarrassment to the state," "criminally inadequate," and so on, were scattered throughout. Few schools escaped his caustic comments, and the administrators of many complained that the review was too hastily done, replete with errors, and "unfair to many small and worthy schools."[13]

Like it or not, the Flexner report had a huge and immediate impact on North American medical education. Its repercussions were felt throughout the country and ultimately served several purposes, many of which can still be seen today. One of the most striking changes wrought by Flexner's review was his belief that all medical schools should be affiliated with major universities. This practice was the norm in the well-respected schools of England, Germany, and France, and although some North American schools had adopted this approach, Flexner postulated that these should serve as the models for all medical schools. Thus, as he investigated each medical school he would write in his report of the need to open unaffiliated hospital wards to teaching and the need of universities to "secure sufficient funds on their side to employ teachers who are devoted to clinical science."[14]

The report also noted the excessive number of physicians in this country, and was ultimately responsible for reducing this number. The ratio of physicians to people in the United States was four to five times greater than in Europe, and many doctors were not as well trained as their counterparts there. Although one reason for the higher ratio was the lower population density in the United States due to the predominance of the agrarian way of life, nonetheless the number was too high. Furthermore, many of the U.S. physicians were underemployed and made very low wages. In his introduction to the report, Henry S. Pritchett, then president of the Carnegie Foundation, complained about "the vast army" of physicians churned out by the plethora of medical schools. He believed, like many in organized medicine, that by reducing the supply of doctors, physicians could not only make a better livelihood, they could better serve the citizenry.

Flexner's study was not the sole source of inspiration for the massive changes that took place in medical education in the early twentieth century. Educators, government officials and those in the medical community were well aware of the need for higher standards for medical schools. But Flexner's work increased awareness of all that needed to be done.

The Flexner Report and Alabama

The impact of the Flexner report was felt immediately in Alabama. When Flexner made his rounds in 1909, the first two schools he visited were the Birmingham Medical College and the Medical Department of the University of Alabama (in Mobile). Flexner's evaluation of both schools was given under the tactful heading "General Considerations." He reported that "really satisfactory medical education is not now to be had in Alabama." He therefore recommended that the Mobile school be moved to Tuscaloosa so that it would be an integral part of the university and that it be reduced from a four-year institution to a two-year basic sciences program. Flexner also proposed, in a recommendation that would prove prophetic, the development of a complete medical school in Birmingham under the control of the university at a later date.

Flexner's work in Alabama was made easier by the fact that both schools had opted to undergo reviews by the AMA's Council on Medical Education in 1907 and as such, had received passing grades (Mobile was rated as "A," Birmingham was given a "B"). After the 1907 reviews, both colleges worked hard to improve curricula and increase their faculty, but "the changes were too late and too little."[15]

Flexner's criticism of both programs did ultimately serve as a powerful impetus to improvement. The Birmingham school, eager to reform its tarnished reputation, began an ambitious fundraising effort that would pay for numerous reforms, including renovations to the main facility and the addition of laboratories, a library, a museum, and a pathology building. When, in 1911, Birmingham school officials approached the state legislature requesting half of the $5,000 appropriation ordinarily given to the Mobile school, a compromise was worked out. The Birmingham Medical College would be given to the University of Alabama (UA) and reorganized as a graduate school of medicine. Its purpose was to train both specialists and general physicians in the latest medical developments, which it began to do in 1913. However, the failure of the state to provide funds for the graduate school resulted in its closure in 1915.

The medical school in Mobile was also seeing its share of hard times. State funding for the school was still very low, but the school's administration strove to make improvements and increase the entrance requirements. However, with enrollment shrinking and a painful lack of endowment and financial support from the state, the Mobile school was in trouble. By 1919 UA president George Denny requested that the AMA Council on Medical Education reevaluate the school in Mobile in an attempt to have the school moved to Tuscaloosa. The review by the Council resulted in a recommendation that the school be moved to Tuscaloosa, which was endorsed by the trustees of the University and implemented in 1920.

Medical Education Arrives in Tuscaloosa

When the equipment in Mobile's medical school was put on railroad cars and transported to Tuscaloosa in the summer of 1920, there was great resentment in the city of Mobile. Indeed, it would be fifty-three years before another medical school would be established in its place.

In Tuscaloosa, home to the state's largest university, the new two-year school was welcomed with great fanfare. The program was placed under the administrative control of Denny, who asked Dr. Clyde Brooks to serve as new dean of the Medical Department of Alabama. Brooks, a native of Paris, Missouri, was trained at Rush Medical College in Chicago and then held teaching positions at various universities before coming to Tuscaloosa in 1920. A professor of physiology and pharmacology, he served as dean for eight years. He continued to teach until 1931 when he left Alabama to join the new medical school at Louisiana State University at New Orleans.

The new arrangements were very much to the liking of President

Denny, an ambitious and popular administrator who was educated in Virginia and served as president at Washington and Lee University before joining UA in 1912. Denny aspired to "build an institution of which the entire state would be proud" and guided the university through a period of extraordinary growth. During his twenty-four years as president, he added six major new programs to the institution, including the new two-year medical department.[16]

A key figure in the early years of the two-year program in Tuscaloosa was Dr. Stuart Graves, who was appointed dean of the medical school in 1928. A native of New York, Graves received his medical degree from Syracuse University in 1911. He taught at the School of Medicine at the University of Louisville before being made dean of that school in 1922, a position he held until accepting the post in Tuscaloosa. In Alabama, Graves became known as an accomplished administrator who worked diligently to build the reputation of the program.

The new school, consisting only of a basic sciences program, was the only medical education offered in the state: its graduates therefore had to go out of state to complete their medical education. Many in the state at this time, including Denny, immediately aspired to expand the program to a complete four-year medical school. The need was obvious: many of those who left the state to complete their education elsewhere would "never return to the people that need them."[17]

In 1922 the leaders at UA moved their program into the newly constructed Nott Hall, named for Dr. Josiah Clark Nott. Located prominently on Sixth Avenue on the campus's central quadrangle, the modern three-story building consisted of laboratories, classrooms and administrative offices. Nott Hall was part of a major building program by Denny, who orchestrated the completion of fourteen major buildings on campus, plus a new football stadium, during his tenure.

The first class of students in Tuscaloosa, which numbered twenty-six, entered in 1920. Because no students were transferred from the Mobile campus, there was no class of second-year students. Many students opted to take so-called combined courses that lasted for four years; this enabled them to earn a Bachelor of Science degree plus the first two years of medical school during a four-year course of study. These students would then complete the two clinical years of their medical education elsewhere. The number of students who received the baccalaureate degree varied greatly each year, from a low of three to a high of twenty-eight.

Entrance requirements for the school increased steadily as the years went by. Initially, thirty semester hours of college credit were required for admission, but by 1930, this number was increased to seventy semester hours. By 1938, this number was increased to ninety semester hours, in spite of the fact that the Depression had constrained the number of students who could afford to attend college.

Many notable faculty members served the program over the course of its twenty-five-year existence. Dr. George T. Pack, for example, was hired by Dean Brooks to teach pathology. A graduate of Yale, he eventually became associate dean of the medical school from 1923–26 before moving to New York, where he became one of the leading cancer surgeons in the country, well known for his bold and radical attacks on cancer. He became a leading figure at New York Cancer Hospital, which later evolved into the Memorial Sloan-Kettering Cancer Center.

Dr. James S. McLester also made significant contributions to the program as a faculty member, serving the university from 1920 until 1945. McLester was interested in clinical nutrition and wrote several books about the role of diet in health and disease. Among his many accomplishments was his role in integrating nutrition into the teaching of medicine. In 1945 he was appointed professor of medicine and chairman of the department at the new four-year medical school in Birmingham, a position he held until his retirement in 1949.

Dr. Allan Walker Blair also served the university's early medical school as assistant professor of pathology and bacteriology from 1929–34. A native of Saskatchewan, Canada, Blair made a name for himself in medical circles when he conducted a study on the black widow spider by allowing one to bite him. His meticulously recorded response, published in the *Archives of Internal Medicine,* established the standard clinical description of the poorly recognized envenomization—and almost cost him his life.[18]

Admissions during the twenty-five years of the program averaged fifty-five per year. Initially, most of these came from Alabama, and the students went on to complete their education at nearby southern medical schools. However, as the reputation of the school spread, a few students went on to prestigious schools in the Northeast and Midwest. Washington University in St. Louis, Missouri, for example, attracted one or two students per year and others went on to such institutions as Harvard, Northwestern, Tulane, and the University of Pennsylvania.

Dr. Gordon King, a prominent member of the surgical staff at Druid

City Hospital in the 1950s and beyond, completed the two-year program before going on to Tulane. He mentioned the excellent reputation that the school had built over the years, noting that those who left the UA medical program went on to excel in their junior and senior years of medical school. He went on to say, "There was not a single failure, as far as I know, of a person [who left UA and] started the third year somewhere else that didn't do well and graduate. We ran circles around the other schools."

Admissions at Tuscaloosa dramatically increased during World War II. During this time U.S. medical schools took a direct role in the war effort by agreeing to help increase the supply of doctors: the nation desperately needed more physicians for the armed forces. Accordingly, the AAMC recommended that medical schools admit a new class every nine months, thus shortening the four-year medical school education to thirty-six months. In spite of some concerns about the quality of these accelerated programs, almost all schools complied.[19] As a result, almost 25,000 doctors were graduated during the war.

The program, however short-lived, proved to be a success. In the twenty-five years the UA offered the two-year program, 1,113 students completed it, including nineteen women. Of those who finished the program in Tuscaloosa, only one percent failed to complete their medical educations. As the years went by, that ratio was reduced to one half of one percent.

Many distinguished physicians had their start in medical school in this program and many returned to Alabama to practice after completing medical school at first-rate institutions across the country. Medical care in Alabama would have been poorer had it not been for these physicians, especially during World War II. Prewar mobilization followed by the diversion of virtually all medical school graduates for five years created a huge shortage of doctors to serve the home front.

The Push for a Four-Year Medical School

In spite of the many successes being witnessed on the Tuscaloosa campus, many from both the public and private sector were dissatisfied with the state of medical education in Alabama, and they began to lobby for the development of a four-year medical school. Interest in such a program had begun almost immediately after the closing of the Mobile campus.

To many the two-year program in Tuscaloosa was simply not enough if Alabama was going to educate its own doctors. The university newspaper lamented that lack of opportunities in medical education in the state:

> Medicine is the one important profession in which Alabama does not now provide a complete education for its own young people. Not only does a large proportion of her native sons and daughters, who are forced to go elsewhere for their medical education, never return to the service of their State, but those same young people carry away enough cash every year to pay the interest on a principal sum sufficient to build and equip and maintain a four-year school and teaching hospital and leave enough to retire the principal, if borrowed, within a comparatively short term of years.[20]

Among those who agitated for change in Alabama was Col. Hopson Owen Murfee, a native of Prattville, Alabama, and an educator, who believed that more needed to be done to improve Alabama's medical facilities. To this end, he organized an influential citizen's advisory group, the Alabama Citizens' Committee, in 1936, which was instrumental in making key changes to the state's medical services, particularly in the mental health institutions of the state. He worked tirelessly to ensure that the committee's work would be seriously considered by all appropriate leaders in state government, the public and private colleges and universities in the state, and leading figures in medical education in the country.

In 1938 Governor Bibb Graves charged Murfee with the task of inspecting the leading mental hospitals, medical centers, and schools in the United States and Canada. The most urgent emphasis was on the needs of the mentally ill in Alabama. But his charge was expanded to include a study of the needs for medical education, a state medical center associated with a new medical school, and the development of state-wide medical centers that could be funded by federal, state, and local funds.

The members of the committee envisioned that several of these health centers would become sites for clinical medical education, the third and fourth years of medical school. This plan would enable the base campus to enroll larger numbers of students for their basic science years, after which time they would move on to the branch campuses for the more expensive and time-consuming clinical years. By then, the concept of learning by doing, in which the students' major experience was gained at the bedside of patients, was well established in medical schools in this country.

After addressing the issues of mental health in Alabama and assuring a million-dollar appropriation to address the state's immediate needs in this area, the committee addressed a much larger task. The group set to work studying what was necessary to build a four-year medical school in the state, soliciting assistance and opinions from some of the greatest medical educators of the day. Murfee solicited recommendations from deans and presidents of many prominent universities with medical schools, as well as from Abraham Flexner, who had become the director of the Institute for Advanced Studies at Princeton. These eminent physicians and educators urged that the medical school in Alabama be established in proximity to the university.

UA president Denny was strongly behind the idea of developing a four-year medical school, and in 1930 he recommended that the university's board of trustees commit itself to building the program as its next major project. The alumni of the university endorsed this move in a resolution that referred to "concern for the future of medical education in this State."[21] To this end, Denny invited Dr. Alan Gregg, a nationally recognized leader in medical education, to evaluate the situation as a representative of the Rockefeller Foundation. Gregg's recommendation was that the two-year program be expanded to become a complete medical school in Tuscaloosa.

Dean Graves was instrumental in helping to create the public desire and public interest that would eventually result in the development of a four-year medical school in 1945.[22] He envisioned a school and a teaching hospital under the authority of the university, with clinics to benefit rural doctors in particular and he presented these proposals to the state medical association and various county associations as well. Graves toured the state promoting this plan and formed two committees, one made up of alumni and the other of members of the state medical association, to help make the four-year school a reality. It was 1943 when the idea caught the attention of then Governor Chauncey Sparks. He announced his intention, as part of his campaign, to build a four-year medical school in Alabama. That year the legislature responded with the passage of Act No. 89, which established the "Medical College of Alabama," later to be known as the University of Alabama School of Medicine (UASOM). Appropriations included $1 million for facilities and equipment and almost $400,000 for maintenance.

The politically charged question of where to locate the new school was still to be decided, however. A committee was appointed by the governor soon after to select a location for the new school. The committee, made up of several physicians and businessmen, considered the most appropriate location. Many argued that the University of Alabama was the rightful location for a medical school: many medical professionals, academics and national authorities, including Gregg, believed the school should be situated in Tuscaloosa. The reality, however, was that the city lacked a large hospital that could serve as a clinical facility—Druid City Hospital had only seventy-five beds—and funds to build a hospital were simply not available. The governor declared that the "building commissions' purpose was to build a medical school, not a hospital."[23] Several public hearings were held and after many months of study, they declared Birmingham to be the most suitable site: no other city could match the facilities available through the Jefferson and Hillman hospitals. Birmingham had offered to let the university have exclusive rights to operate both hospitals, which would make up the nucleus of the new medical center. It was a blow to the city of Tuscaloosa. But with the establishment of the expanded Medical College of Alabama in Birmingham, another phase in medical history in Alabama had begun.

Medical Education Moves to Birmingham

In the summer of 1945, at the end of World War II, the medical school at UA was moved to Birmingham. Truckloads of equipment, books, and specimens were seen winding their way up U.S. Highway 11, then the main route connecting Birmingham and Tuscaloosa. The school was located on a solitary block of real estate in a run-down section of Birmingham, a city well known for its steel industry. The Hillman Hospital and the newer seventeen-story Jefferson Hospital located on South 21st Street housed the new medical program in 1945. Over time the medical school would come to be recognized as a world-class academic health center covering many city blocks.

Dr. Roy R. Kracke, a well-respected hematologist from Hartselle, Alabama, was asked to serve as the first dean of the new medical school. Kracke recognized the possibilities of the new medical school and wasted no time in building the program. By the end of the first year, he had established the School of Dentistry and purchased additional land adjacent to the Jefferson-Hillman complex on which to build the medical center. On October 8, 1945, the first class of students was admitted to the Medical College of Alabama; Birmingham's place in the world of academic medicine was about to be established.

2

Bringing Medical Education Back to Tuscaloosa

The decade of the 1960s was a turbulent time in medical education in the United States as the field underwent breathtaking growth and development. Medical school curricula were revised, faculties grew, enrollments were expanded, and philosophies shifted. These changes were largely fueled by technological advances, combined with an expansion in the United States of higher education and science in general, brought on in large measure by a huge infusion of federal dollars. Almost overnight, medical schools and their affiliated teaching hospitals became much larger and more complex institutions, operating in a world that was similarly large and complicated.[24]

A Changing Emphasis

Although the primary missions of the nation's medical schools—research, teaching, and patient care—had changed very little over time, their emphasis changed a great deal after World War II. One strong trend that emerged after the war was an increased focus on laboratory and clinical research. By the 1950s the National Institutes of Health (NIH) and other federal agencies were allocating massive amounts of money for research: by 1960 federal support of medical research had reached $1.5 billion, a 100-fold increase since 1940. NIH alone contributed more than $1.3 million in 1960, a number that would triple in the next decade. Accordingly, most academic medical centers wanted to partake of this newfound wealth. Likewise, with the passage of the Medicare and Medicaid Acts of 1965, which provided health insurance for the aged and poor respectively, the emphasis on patient care surged. The resulting clinical revenue was huge and allowed these centers to greatly expand their physical facilities and faculties and to raise faculty salaries. As medical schools turned their attention to research and patient care, teaching lagged behind and medical students became their "forgotten members."[25]

The 1960s also saw the publication of three widely distributed reports that would color the nation's approach to medical education for many years to come. The Millis report (sponsored by the AMA), the Coggeshall report (sponsored by the AAMC) and the Willard report (sponsored by the AMA's Council on Medical Education) identified changes that were needed in the nation's approach to teaching health professionals. All three commissions agreed that the American medical education process was placing too much emphasis on research, specialization, and subspecialization—and too little on the training of primary care physicians.

In particular, it was the Millis report of 1966, written by Dr. John Millis, president of Western Reserve University in Ohio, which so pointedly addressed the crisis in primary care. In fact, the commission devoted an entire chapter to the need for physicians who would practice comprehensive care. The report's authors lamented the decline of general practitioners, pointing out that the few training programs that existed for general practitioners failed to address the full array of knowledge required for such a physician. The report conceived of programs that went beyond "the knowledge of organs, systems and techniques" and instead focused on "the whole man who lives in a complex social setting."[26] Furthermore, continued the report's authors, "If the full range of medical competence is to be made effectively and efficiently available, it is mandatory that means be found to increase the supply of physicians willing and properly trained to serve in this comprehensive role." The report went on to detail the various aspects of needed changes in the medical school curriculum, the change from total emphasis on hospital patients to office patients, where continuing care can be practiced. Furthermore, the report's authors spoke of the need to establish the comprehensive physician as an equal in the medical hierarchy.

The Coggeshall report, officially entitled "Planning for Medical Progress through Education," was released in 1965 and provided an in-depth analysis of medical education at the time. The leader in this effort was Dr. Lowell T. Coggeshall, vice president at the University of Chicago. He and the other members of the committee spoke of the many trends in medical education, their implications, and the recommendations for the future, including a proposal to improve the development of family practice. The report's authors made numerous specific recommendations, including the reorganization and enlargement of the AAMC, as well as its relocation to Washington, D.C. These changes would eventually lead to that organization's establishment as a major resource to the federal government in matters related to medical education and its hearty endorsement of a major expansion of medical school class sizes in many of America's medical schools.

The third report published during this time was produced by the Ad Hoc Committee on Education for Family Practice, published in 1966. The influential committee was chaired by Dr. William R. Willard, dean of the medical school at the University of Kentucky who later was appointed dean of the new medical education program at UA in Tuscaloosa. Entitled "Meeting the Challenge of Family Practice," the report advocated a new field to be called "family practice" designed to help provide comprehensive personal health care in the increasingly complex and specialized world of medicine. The report defined the family physician: one who would serve as the first contact with the patient and provide "a means of entry into the health care system."[27] This doctor would look beyond the individual to the family and community and assume responsibility for the patient's total health care needs. The report also outlined a proposal for educating these new professionals, arguing for rigorous training in comprehensive care, "an objective quite different from that in more limited specialties where expertise is sought in a narrower area."[28] The last key feature of the report was a plea for board certification for the group, which they believed would provide status for the field and reward for those who were thus trained. The committee's recommendations were based on a conviction that more needed to be done to increase the supply of well-trained family physicians. Implementation of these concepts beginning in the 1970s in fact ultimately provided more general physicians, particularly for small towns and rural areas. Furthermore, publication of this report accelerated the efforts of the family physicians, medical educators, and state and federal legislators to create the new specialty. The American Board of Family Practice was established in 1969.

Also of consequence during the 1960s was the publication of a seminal paper by K. W. Deuschle and F. Eberson of the University of Kentucky, where Willard had established one of the first departments of Community Medicine in the country. Writing in the *Journal of Medical Education*, they described an innovative program at the University of Kentucky in

Lexington that exemplified the concepts of community medicine as "a cooperative integrated program of medical and biological disciplines for studying and solving in-depth community health problems."[29] The authors preached the importance of this mission in medicine and advocated the adoption of such an approach for all medical schools. Charles E. Lewis, a well-respected figure in medical education, and his colleague Richard Easton would write from the Center for Community Health and Medical Care at Harvard University, that, as a result of the Deuschle-Eberson article, there was "an epidemic of community health fever" going around.[30]

Outside the medical institutions, other factors were at work that would revolutionize medicine and ultimately, medical education. Increasingly since the Second World War, people were demanding more and better health care. The demand was attributed to many factors: population growth, especially among the aged; increased expectations of individuals; a heightened level of health consciousness by the public; a greater availability of health insurance; and an overall increase in economic prosperity. All contributed to a demand that greatly exceeded the ability of physicians in practice to provide it. The U.S. Public Health Service in 1965 estimated a national shortage of 50,000 physicians. Legislators and the public looked to the medical establishment to solve the crisis, which many believed called for the training of more physicians.

Seeking Medical Progress in Alabama

Much of what was occurring at that time at the national level in medical education was also taking place in the state of Alabama. Many, including those in the medical community, could see the changes that were taking place in the field and they too voiced concern. Vigorous arguments took place concerning the dominance of specialists and the related decline of general practitioners. One person who stirred up interest was Dr. Richard Rutland, president of the state chapter of the American Academy of Family Physicians in 1961–62 and a general practitioner in Fayette, Alabama, a small town located approximately forty miles north of Tuscaloosa. Rutland, a staunch believer in the value of the family doctor, became a vocal advocate for more primary care physicians after witnessing not only a decline in the number of practicing general practitioners, but a noticeable "loss of prestige for the field as a whole."[31] He felt one approach to alleviating the shortage of family physicians, especially in rural areas, was to encourage more students to experience rural family practice while in medical school; he pressed the leadership at the medical school in Birmingham to place greater emphasis on this area. He succeeded in developing Fayette as a preceptor site for Birmingham students who wanted a rural experience, but this proved to be insufficient. Clearly more needed to be done to address the shortage of family physicians.

It was only later, as the demand for more doctors in Alabama grew more clamorous, that the issue would catch the attention of Governor George C. Wallace. And in that lay a solution.

Wallace dominated the political scene in Alabama for many years, serving the first of his three terms from 1962–1966. Essentially a populist, George Wallace developed a national and international reputation as a man who played racial politics to win elections. Although this would enhance Wallace's career and propel him into the national spotlight, the end result was years of violence and economic stagnation for Alabama.

"Alabama's place in the national medical community could not have been lower then it was in the early 1960s," wrote Dr. Clifton Meador, dean of the medical school at UAB from 1968 through 1973, in a letter to the College of Community Health Sciences (CCHS) committee charged with developing this book. "The racial problems were the major cause, as were Wallace's embarrassing national tirades and tactics."

Yet in spite of the negative effects of his policies, Governor Wallace succeeded in delivering many of the improvements he promised, including new highways, increased industrial recruitment, and improved education. His focus on education—primarily the result of his belief that educational opportunities should be readily available to every Alabama citizen—translated to a network of new trade schools, junior colleges, and community colleges. In many ways, it was this thinking, combined with public support for these programs, which led to the creation of the medical education programs in Huntsville and Tuscaloosa, and a complete new medical school in Mobile at the University of South Alabama.

The Commissioning of the Booz, Allen, Hamilton Report

By 1967 the public outcry from Alabama's citizens concerning the doctor shortage had reached a crescendo. It was a cry that the Wallace administration heard and took to heart. In July 1967 the Alabama Legislature commissioned the nationally known Virginia-based consulting firm of Booz, Allen, Hamilton, Inc. to undertake a study of the state's medical manpower needs and to recommend appropriate solutions.

The results of the study confirmed what the public believed about health care in Alabama: the state was suffering from a serious shortage of physicians. The authors of the study reported that according to the AMA and the U.S. Bureau of Census, across the nation there were 144 physicians per 100,000 persons in 1967. In Alabama, that number was only eighty per 100,000 persons—well below the national average—and that ratio was not expected to improve over the next decade. With estimates that the state's population would increase from 3.49 million to 4.5 million by 1985, Alabama was looking at a growing crisis of increasingly limited access to health care.

The report listed numerous reasons for the shortage of physicians, ranging from increased demand by citizens to the movement of doctors from rural areas to metropolitan ones. The report's authors also recorded a dearth of doctors specializing in primary care. New opportunities in clinical subspecialties, research, administration, public health, and teaching were available, thus reducing the number of physicians willing or able to provide comprehensive care. Rapidly expanding technology caused the development of new specialties and subspecialties, and students were often excited by the opportunity to excel in one limited area.

The emphasis in medical schools seemed to be on research and not education, the report stated. In one study covering the period from the early 1950s to 1967, the full-time faculty of medical schools had risen over 400 percent and research expenditures increased by a similar percent. At the same time, enrollment had risen only 27 percent.

The Booz, Allen, Hamilton report also cited another reason for the national shortage of physicians: the geographic maldistribution of doctors. Rural areas do not attract physicians as large cities do. And the movement of physicians to metropolitan areas worsened an already critical problem in the rural areas. In Alabama, as nationally, the physician-to-population ratio for metropolitan areas was almost twice that for non-metropolitan areas. The end result for people in rural Alabama was limited access to physicians of any kind.

The Booz, Allen, Hamilton report also noted that almost three-fourths of the physicians practicing in the state had received their medical degree elsewhere. With the growing demand for physicians nationwide, wrote the authors, Alabama must reduce its reliance on out-of-state physicians.

Several ways to correct these shortcomings were recommended. First was a thorough expansion of medical education in the state to allow for the graduation of more physicians. The report suggested the establishment of clinical sciences programs at both the University of South Alabama in Mobile and the University of Alabama–Huntsville (UAH), where third- and fourth-year medical students, those enrolled in the clinical years of the medical curriculum, could have their entire clinical experience in a community setting, supervised by practicing physicians. The report also recommended the addition of a new basic sciences program at UA in Tuscaloosa, where students could complete the first two years of the medical school curriculum.

The report's authors also suggested that the medical college at Birmingham expand its enrollment, a recommendation that coincided with an endorsement by the AMA that "all medical schools should now accept as a goal the expansion of their collective enrollments to a level that permits all qualified applicants to be admitted."[32] The Booz, Allen, Hamilton report also suggested increasing the number of graduate medical programs in the state, including residencies and internships. They cited studies showing that physicians tend to settle in the general area where they obtained their graduate training.

The results of the report were useful, but they begged a much larger question for the state of Alabama: could such large-scale changes really be wrought in a state that placed so little emphasis on education? In the 1960s Alabama ranked at or near the bottom of all states in most categories of education, including spending per student and teacher salaries. But the report's authors warned that the expansion of medical education was critical if the state was to avoid a future health care crisis. "Obviously, if the number of medical students graduated in Alabama is to be significantly increased," wrote the authors of the report, "major additional income must be identified, regardless of the source or the means used to expand undergraduate medical education."[33]

In spite of concerns about funding these ventures, the state legislature endorsed the Booz, Allen, Hamilton recommendations in 1968, thus providing a crucial spur to the establishment of the medical education programs in Tuscaloosa, Huntsville, and Mobile.

University Takes Action on the Booz, Allen, Hamilton Recommendations

The UA administration under the direction of President Frank A. Rose immediately began to study ways to implement the recommendations of the report. In September 1968 Rose established a task force under the direction of Wayne H. Finley, M.D., Ph.D., a distinguished professor of pediatrics at UAB. Serving on the committee were Dr. Charles T. Moore, assistant vice president for Academic Affairs, Dr. Sydenham Alexander, director of the Student Health Service, Dr. Douglas Jones, interim dean (and later dean) of the College of Arts and Sciences, and Dr. John Burnum, a highly regarded local internist.

Over the next two years, the committee engaged in intense discussion over the form that medical education in Tuscaloosa should take, including the "purpose and character" of such a program. Members of the committee also visited several medical schools representing student-learning models (for example, Brown and Michigan State) and the research-oriented model (Johns Hopkins) in order to determine what elements of these programs might be appropriate for the new UA-based program.

Discussions during this time also speculated on what role the local hospital—then Druid City Hospital, renamed DCH—might play in the medical education program. Founded in 1923 and close to the UA campus on University Boulevard, DCH had grown from a small hospital with only fifty beds to a modern four-hundred-bed facility that had received magazine coverage in both *Life* and *Modern Hospital.* By 1970 DCH was the third largest general hospital in the state and, with additional growth planned, DCH was viewed as an excellent place to train students in a community-hospital setting. UA administrators looked seriously at forming a partnership with the hospital. The idea of using community-based hospitals for medical education had recently grown in popularity. Conventional wisdom was that these new community-based schools in general were more receptive to new approaches in curricula, more sensitive to community health issues and more interested in helping to produce primary care physicians than were academic medical centers. "All of the medical journals ring with the theme of interdigitating some segment of the training of the physicians into a community hospital setting," wrote Burnum in a letter to the UA president in September 1969. The philosophical advantages of such an arrangement, combined with the availability of federal funds for developing model community hospitals, made this a logical route for the new medical education program to take.

Planning for what would become CCHS continued in this vein for several years. The original planners, working with an administration keen to revive medical education in Tuscaloosa, addressed many key elements of the program. Questions about what type of program the university wanted, what faculty and facilities would be needed, and what form of funding would be necessary were all examined in detail. These considerations were made within the context of the recommendations of Booz, Allen, Hamilton and the needs of the state, as well as the nation as it dealt with similar issues.

Mathews Leads Planning at UA

In the midst of this planning period, major changes took place in the governance of the UA system. In January 1969 Dr. Rose, who had presided over the three university campuses for eleven years, announced his plans to leave the university. However, instead of replacing him with a single president for the entire system, the board of trustees named a president for each four-year institution. Dr. Joseph Volker was named as president of UAB, Dr. Benjamin Graves was asked to preside over the Huntsville program, and Dr. David Mathews was promoted from executive vice president to president of UA in Tuscaloosa. This reorganization rendered each institution essentially autonomous.

The appointment of Mathews resulted in a tremendous boost for the planning effort in Tuscaloosa. A native of Grove Hill, Alabama, Mathews was a staunch supporter of medical education. At age thirty-three he was the youngest university president in the nation in 1969. "He had an abiding interest in engaging the university in the problems of the state and in community life," recalled Burnum.[34] Nationally, Mathews became well known as someone who challenged institutions of higher learning to "pursue new ventures in public service."[35]

Mathews wasted little time securing the support he needed from UAB and DCH to build a medical education program in Tuscaloosa. Of special concern was building a cooperative arrangement with the medical school in Birmingham. Those who were involved in the planning acknowledged that the program could not succeed without the cooperation of the administrators of the medical school in Birmingham; however, issues regarding the governance of the program were sometimes contentious.

Also important were relations with DCH. In the midst of the planning, the doctors at DCH voiced opposition to the program. Their objection to the proposed program grew in part from an experience at Jefferson-Hillman Hospital in Birmingham, which had been taken over by UAB as a teaching hospital in 1945. Full-time academic physicians had eased out long-term staffers as the teaching program grew, and the medical and surgical staff at DCH feared they would meet a similar fate.

Dr. Gordon King, a prominent member of the hospital staff, was instrumental in gaining the support of the medical staff at DCH. "At the time we had a rather small staff, a very close-knit group, a group that was pretty set in their ways and opinionated about things and [they did] not welcome a whole lot of change," he said in an interview. "So we had a lot of groundwork to do, a lot of convincing to do about what medical education meant to the staff and Tuscaloosa County. We had to convince a lot of the people who had been here that it was in the interest of the patients of Tuscaloosa to have an educational program and for the medical and surgical staff to serve as role models."

Mathews, King, and Burnum worked to allay the fears of those at the hospital and by March 1970, the hospital agreed to earmark up to $100,000 for a teaching program. The decision was heralded in Tuscaloosa where the newspaper announced that the DCH board of trustees had agreed to build a "model hospital" and eventually establish a clinical teaching program.[36] Although the support of the hospital would waver periodically as the program evolved, DCH had officially committed to the program.

During the same period, Mathews also undertook a vigorous effort to secure the cooperation of the business leaders of the community and the state's legislators, support that would be important in the years to come. Mathews later referred to the importance of this multifaceted effort, indicating they would "talk to anyone who would listen about the unique mission of the College." Later, Burnum would credit Mathews as being the cornerstone of the medical education program in Tuscaloosa, referring to Mathew's "steadfast" leadership, energy, and optimism that made the program a reality.

Burnum himself would also play a major role in the formation of the college. A native of Tuscaloosa, with a medical degree from Harvard Medical School, Burnum had practiced internal medicine in his hometown since 1954. With an impressive clinical research record, he had gained the respect of many in the community and at the medical school in Birmingham. In September 1969 he was asked to serve as Mathew's special assistant for Medical Affairs for the university. At the same time he was also asked to serve DCH as the director of Medical Education, thus becoming a vital link between the community physicians, the hospital, UAB, and UA.

Solidifying the Program

By August 1970, with considerable input from the administration in Birmingham, the university had decided on the fundamentals of their program. First, it was agreed that Tuscaloosa should develop a clinical education program, that is, the last two years of undergraduate medical education, instead of the first two years of medical school as had been originally recommended. This plan proved to be more acceptable to the faculty and administrators in Birmingham, where some perceived that the basic sciences were weak on the UA campus. Furthermore, the program in Birmingham already needed additional faculty and space; it would be more efficient to build on the existing departments and programs.

The decision to include third- and fourth-year students for their clinical training in Tuscaloosa—instead of first- and second-year students—was also much more popular at DCH. King referred to this decision as marking a "turning point" in the level of acceptance by the DCH medical staff: he noted that the staff could much more easily imagine "teaching these kids surgical principles, urology and that sort of thing, rather than amino acids."

The planners also agreed to develop a residency program in family practice. This decision helped alleviate some concerns at DCH, where some staff members perceived residencies in other specialties as a threat. Furthermore, there was general agreement that family practice residents could be useful in caring for the indigent patients who often sought care at the hospital emergency room, and in assisting staff physicians in caring for many patients, both public and private.

Thirdly, it was decided that the new school would be led by its own dean, who would report to both the vice president for Health Affairs on the UAB campus and the UA president in Tuscaloosa. This dual reporting structure made perfect sense at the time but would later cause difficulties between the two organizations.

The next step was to secure funding for the new college. Mathews urged local doctors, hospital administrators, and the board of the hospital to write to Governor-elect Wallace stressing the need for a medical education program in Tuscaloosa that was focused on training doctors for small towns and rural areas. A conference was also organized to discuss the exploration of federal funding. Planning proceeded reasonably well in this vein. A curriculum that stressed comprehensive patient care in a community setting was discussed, and a committee was formed to locate a dean for the new program.

In March 1971, however, the program ran into a roadblock that almost spelled its end. At a clinical medicine symposium held in Tuscaloosa, UAB administrators suddenly and publicly withdrew their support. Word that a four-year medical school would be built at the University of South Alabama in Mobile had just reached UAB, and concerns about costs abounded. Clearly, establishment of a separate medical school in Mobile would far exceed the costs of the UAB extensions to include new programs in Tuscaloosa, Huntsville, and perhaps other sites.

A statement by Dean Clifton K. Meador was read by Dr. John M. Packard, who was then director of the Alabama Regional Medical program in Birmingham:

> It is now apparent that a second four-year medical school will be created in Mobile, with additional heavy expense in duplicating the costly basic science courses. The State of Alabama will have trouble funding two full medical schools. In my opinion, it will be impossible to fund any additional medical schools in the state, even the two-year schools suggested for Tuscaloosa and Huntsville. I am therefore withdrawing my proposal.

Even today, Meador stands by this decision. "With the plight of public schools in the state at the elementary level, combined with the state being somewhere near the bottom in money for education, it made no sense to dump additional money into medical education, even at UAB. The idea of starting three new medical schools in one of the nation's poorest states was ridiculous," wrote Meador.

On the UA campus, Mathews and Burnum were also seeking immediate reassurance and within days met with Governor Wallace to seek other sources of funding. This consultation, in addition to a great deal of public support for the program, led the governor to call a special session of the Legislature. A new state senator, Richard Shelby, introduced the legislation that would provide $4 million in capital funds for the proposed clinical programs in Tuscaloosa and Huntsville. These funds, which were approved, were combined with the $435,000 in planning money that had been appropriated in the spring, and provided the crucial infusion of money needed to get the program off the ground. Medical education in Tuscaloosa was on its way.

3
Laying the Groundwork for CCHS

The unexpected appropriation of funds in May 1971 for the two-year programs in Huntsville and Tuscaloosa gave UA a decidedly positive push. Suddenly, after years of hard work and numerous false starts and disappointments, the university had the financial backing it needed to get the program underway. It must have seemed to the planners of the program that this support would never come. Yet, as Dr. Richard Rutland would later observe, "George Wallace was true to his word" and that year, in spite of a noticeable lack of support from officials at UASOM, medical education in Tuscaloosa became a reality.[37]

Identifying a Dean

Although a great deal of work had been done in the preceding years planning the role of the school and discussing possible faculty and facilities, there was now a pressing need to get personnel committed to the program, most notably a dean for the new college. Attention immediately focused on one individual, Dr. William R. Willard, who was by then recognized as a pioneer in the definition and sanctioning of family medicine in the United States.

At the time Willard was serving as the special assistant to the president for medical affairs at the University of Kentucky, where he had played a pivotal role in the development of the medical school in 1956. As the founding dean of the College of Medicine there, Willard had a reputation for innovative approaches to medical education, enthusiasm, and hard work; he appeared to be an excellent match for the needs of the state of Alabama.

In 1971, as UA was formalizing its medical education program, Willard was quickly approaching mandatory retirement age at Kentucky, and he and his wife were looking at various options for life after retirement. One avocation that appealed to them was catfish farming, and they soon began visiting catfish farms and processors in Texas, Louisiana, Mississippi, and Alabama.

It was during this time that Willard was contacted by Dr. Howard Gundy, the academic vice president at UA and a longtime friend with whom Willard had worked at the University of Syracuse. Gundy reported that UA officials were interested in talking to him about the leadership of an innovative new program in community medical education. Thus, Willard was invited to Tuscaloosa.

During Willard's visit to Tuscaloosa, the president of UA at Tuscaloosa, Dr. David Mathews, called on Victor Poole, a politically well-connected businessman with a long-standing commitment to improving public education, and asked him to host Willard for a visit to nearby Moundville, where Poole resided. UA administrators had learned of Willard's interest in catfish farming, and Poole was able to convince him that Moundville, a community of one thousand people located only fourteen miles from the UA campus, would be an excellent place to set up shop. This, combined with an opportunity to develop an innovative medical education program, must have looked irresistible to Dr. Willard.

Later, he would speak of his decision to join UA. "I've always been interested in the development process. But my hope was not just to train family physicians and other personnel for Alabama. I hoped we could motivate students to provide humane and personalized comprehensive medical care as primary care physicians and to engage in significant public service," he said.[38]

This, then, was the vision of William Willard in 1972 when he retired from the University of Kentucky to join UA in July of that year. In him the university found an experienced medical school administrator who could potentially transform medical education in Alabama.

An Experienced Leader

Willard was born in 1908 and grew up in Seattle, Washington. He went to Yale University, where he earned his undergraduate degree in 1931 and his medical degree in 1934. After two years of residency in pediatrics, one at Johns Hopkins and the other at Strong Memorial Hospital in Rochester, New York, Willard returned to Yale where he earned a doctorate in public health in 1937. He then joined the Maryland State Health Department where he worked for seven years. Later, he would describe these years as being pivotal as he formulated his ideas about the need for a productive alliance between medicine and public health.

In 1944 Willard enlisted in the military and was promptly sent to Korea, where he spent two years working as acting director of public health and welfare for military personnel stationed in Seoul. Upon his return, although urged to rejoin the health department of Maryland, Willard joined the faculty at his alma mater, where he rapidly rose through the ranks of academia and became assistant dean in charge of postgraduate medical education in 1948.

By the age of forty-three, Willard had amassed an impressive array of credentials that acknowledged his productivity, ambition, and vision. His unique combination of experience, philosophy, and personal style brought him wide respect, both at Yale and in other academic medical circles.

In 1951 Willard was offered the position of dean at the State University of New York (SUNY) Upstate Medical Center in Syracuse. Only one year before, SUNY assumed responsibility for the medical school, and Willard viewed the position as an opportunity to put many of his views about medical education into practice. One of the major thrusts at Syracuse was recruiting professionals into his newly designed venture, people who would help him develop the novel program. He added to his staff, not just professionals in the traditional departments, but several in nontraditional ones as well—hiring faculty members specializing in health economics, medical ethics, and behavioral science. This was done in accordance with Willard's determined view that medical education needed to be expanded beyond the biological factors that affect health status to the social, cultural, and behavioral factors that also play a crucial role. This initiative added a new dimension to medical education and broadened the scope of the students who went through the program.

In the five years that Willard spent at Syracuse, he had many accomplishments to his name. Yet, in spite of his success and his excellent reputation, Willard was frustrated by his lack of autonomy in the SUNY system: he was three steps removed from the decision-making process for capital expenditure and operating budgets, and he felt this stymied the progress of the medical school. It is not difficult to understand his desire to continue his work in a more receptive environment.

That opportunity came in the form of an offer from the University of

Kentucky in 1956. In Lexington, Willard was not only asked to be founding dean, but "chief architect" of a new medical program. His charge was to design, build, staff, and direct an entirely new medical school, dental school, nursing school, and hospital. Here again, he pursued an ambitious program that integrated behavioral science, community health, and public health practices into the traditional medical education curriculum.[39] Later, this novel endeavor would be recognized as invaluable to the entire field. In a tribute to Willard in 1979, U.S. Assistant Secretary for Health and Surgeon General Julius B. Richmond would remark that Willard's work at Kentucky was "a truly pioneering enterprise, one which would change the course of medical education and health services in our country."[40]

In 1972 Willard also received recognition from AAMC in the form of the Flexner Award, the highest award given by the association. It was this experience and prestige, combined with sixteen productive years at Kentucky, that he brought to UA. His firmly held beliefs about medical education and the future of medicine would once again be applied to a new program, in a new state.

Willard's Philosophy

With forty-three years in the medical field, Willard had strong opinions on the shape that medical education should take, and these were reflected immediately in Tuscaloosa's newly formed medical education program. As founding dean of the college, his philosophy shaped the beginnings of the program, and the faculty he recruited reflected those ideals. Even today, evidence of his profound influence can be seen in the CCHS program.

He had a vision for the program since its inception. Dr. Sandral Hullett, an early resident in the Tuscaloosa program, recalls attending barbecues at Willard's home in Moundville where he would gather the students and residents around him and expound his vision for the college.

"He wanted this to be an institution that would reach out to the surrounding areas and develop providers and improve the health status in those areas and be a resource in those areas. He really had a big ambition for studying the communities and helping them improve themselves," she explained in an interview.

Health care for Willard went beyond the individual: individuals make up families and families make up communities. Willard was able to see beyond the narrow view of so many physicians who, as he stated in a commencement speech, had "no time, no interest and little to no training for helping to solve the larger problem of the health and medical care needs of the community as a whole."[41] In Willard's view, this problem had been aggravated by the trend toward specialization and subspecialization and away from personalized, humane care.

Much of Willard's philosophy became crystallized during his time as chairman of the Ad Hoc Committee on Education for Family Practice. Here, Willard and his fellow committee members studied the American medical educational process and concluded that the traditional programs were placing far too much emphasis on research and specialization. The result was too little training of personal primary care physicians. "The fact remains," lamented the authors of the report, "that virtually no physicians are being trained specifically for careers in family practice."[42] At Alabama, Willard hoped to change that.

Setting Priorities

The job of developing the medical education program in Tuscaloosa was formidable. The situation at the state level was abysmal: the state was once again strapped for cash and the financial resources needed for this venture were still frustratingly scarce. Likewise, support for the program was also weak. Many important groups, including DCH and UAB, were ambivalent about the proposed medical program in Tuscaloosa. Developing a program "from scratch," as Willard knew from Kentucky, took a great deal of planning. Although years of groundwork had already been laid, much needed to be done: a new residency program had to be developed, facilities for teaching and administration had to be built, and soon, medical students would arrive and need to be trained. In addition, there were the community components that Willard hoped to add to the program.

During his first few months at UA, he met with medical school administrators in Birmingham, with the medical staff at DCH, with legislators, and with many local physicians. The new college could not function without the cooperation of these groups, but Willard was optimistic that people would "come around."

In his first meeting with the medical staff at DCH in the summer of

1972, Willard sought concurrence with the plans that were being formulated. He carefully outlined the vision for the program: a clinical training program for medical students, a family practice residency, continuing education programs, and eventually, a network of primary care centers that would contribute badly needed medical services to the state. The hospital had little experience with medical education, and Willard described his vision of the relationship between DCH and the college. He foresaw a cooperative, mutually beneficial affiliation that would be formed in the interest of medical education, for the good of both organizations and the surrounding community.

But the hospital staff was more resistant than Willard had anticipated. In fact, it was announced at the meeting, the hospital did not intend to finance any aspect of the new program. Hospital administrator D. O. McClusky stated that DCH viewed medical education as the state's responsibility. Willard, although dismayed, accepted the situation, thinking that later "if the program was successful and the residents proved to be useful to the medical staff in Tuscaloosa, the attitude would change."[43]

With help from Mathews and Mr. Richard Thigpen, a law professor and the executive assistant to the president, the new dean also spent a great deal of time drumming up support in the community. All three men met regularly with community leaders and were able to obtain support and much needed funding from some of the larger industries in town, including the Tuscaloosa News, B. F. Goodrich, the Tuscaloosa County Commission, the First National Bank of Tuscaloosa, and the City National Bank of Tuscaloosa. Later, in an effort to organize the support of these community groups, they formed the Lister Hill Society in 1975 with Dr. William Anderson, a radiologist and UA alumnus, as president. This group, named for the state's former senior senator, a major supporter of health programs in Alabama, offered individuals and companies a way to contribute to the college in an attempt to provide improved health care to the state. Over the next three decades, local business leaders proved to be very supportive of the program.

During that first summer, as plans for the new program developed, the need for a distinctive name became apparent. Mathews was the one who suggested the College of Community Health Sciences (CCHS). The name suited Willard, as it appealed to his vision of serving the various outlying rural communities of the state and helping them address their health care problems. The name was officially adopted in the summer of 1972, and the college became a recognized branch campus of UASOM. Together, the medical campuses at Birmingham, Huntsville, and Tuscaloosa would be designated as the University of Alabama School of Medicine Education Program, or UASMEP.

But a program that is little more than an idea, a name, and a leader cannot offer much, and Willard endeavored to forge an organization that would bring medical education back to Tuscaloosa and the communities in need of health care. Accordingly, he turned to the task of hiring his staff, people with the energy and enthusiasm needed to get this ambitious program off the ground.

Recruiting the Initial Staff

Recruiting to the CCHS program, as it turns out, was an arduous task that consumed much of Willard's time and energy for several years. One of the biggest factors was the terrible national image that Alabama had garnered during the racial turmoil of the 1960s. Alabama's reputation for racial conflict and violence placed increased pressure on all types of recruitment in the state.[44] Another disadvantage for Willard was the lack of family physicians in the country—the specialty was quite new and competition was fierce for those who had entered the field.

But the new dean persevered: much had to be done before the campus could welcome students or residents, and Willard needed qualified help. Willard's initial staffing plan was to hire a small nucleus of generalists in each major specialty as full-time faculty and then to supplement their work with local practicing physicians who might be persuaded to volunteer their services.

Dean Willard's first hire was Carolyn Watson as his executive secretary, who was to spend the next ten years working for CCHS. Watson played a key role in keeping the dean's office running, as Willard was often away on recruiting trips in the early years. She was soon joined by Dr. Bobby Moore from the university's biology department, who would handle the administrative details of setting up the new medical education program. Moore had been involved in advising premedical students and agreed to join CCHS full-time as the assistant dean for Administration in October 1972. Moore handled the evolving college's budgetary matters and served as the liaison with the architects that were hired by the university as part of the CCHS building program.

Dr. John Packard, an internist and cardiologist, was hired to serve as the associate dean for Clinical Affairs. Packard, recruited from the Alabama Regional Medical Program in Birmingham and much admired by Willard, was asked to develop the undergraduate program as coordinator of educational programs for the college. In this capacity he would also handle the process of helping the college acquire accreditation, a large and complex task that loomed ahead.

Another addition to the staff was Dr. William Hubbard, hired in May 1973 from Daytona Beach, Florida, where he directed a small family practice residency. Willard asked him to serve as the director of the college's residency program. Although he stayed at Tuscaloosa for only a short time, Hubbard played a crucial role in writing the application for the approval of the family practice residency program, which was provisionally approved by the AMA in September 1973.

Willard's next chore was to recruit physicians to help teach in the program. He started in Fayette, where he met and persuaded Dr. Richard Rutland to join the faculty on a part-time basis. Rutland had been a vocal advocate for the training of more family physicians in the state and felt obliged to be of service to the college. However, Rutland felt torn between his obligations in Fayette and therefore could only commit to come to Tuscaloosa two days each week.

Willard then traveled about the state looking for other faculty members and found Dr. Riley Lumpkin from Enterprise. Willard would later write of Lumpkin that he was "well received in Tuscaloosa, unfailingly cheerful and always popular."[45] Lumpkin was hired as the director of the clinic, to be called the Family Practice Center. He went on to work for the college for twenty-six years, serving as interim dean after Willard's retirement in 1979.

Dr. William deShazo was the next addition to the CCHS staff; he was recruited out of the university's Student Health Service. He had been a general practitioner in south Alabama and had served on the board of the University of South Alabama at the time of its founding, and Willard thought he would make a good addition to the growing team. "With Dr. deShazo, who was a forceful individual with an outgoing personality, we had at least the nucleus of family physicians," Willard later wrote.[46]

The next two additions to the faculty would be Dr. David Hefelfinger, a pediatrician from Pensacola, Florida, and Dr. Jerry Davis, a Tuscaloosa-based pediatrician. They both joined CCHS in early 1974, and Hefelfinger was appointed head of pediatrics. Hefelfinger, born in New Jersey, received both his baccalaureate and medical degrees at the University of North Carolina in Chapel Hill. He then completed his residency training in pediatrics at Vanderbilt University Hospital in Nashville and the University of Texas Medical Branch in Galveston, where he was chief resident. After serving several years in the military, he entered private practice in Florida in 1971. He moved to Tuscaloosa to take the faculty position at CCHS and went on to serve the college for more than twenty-five years before retiring.

Several area family practitioners from throughout the state agreed to serve as instructors at least on a part-time basis, and they proved to be invaluable during the early years of the program when the college had a small faculty. Among them were Dr. Bill Owings of Centreville, Dr. Leroy Holt of Bessemer, Dr. Rucker Staggers of Eutaw, Dr. Henry C. "Moon" Mullins of Mobile, and Dr. Willis Israel of Wedowee.

The next issue for the new college was in the area of surgery. In the early 1970s Tuscaloosa had many general surgeons, and they openly resisted the idea of a full-time surgeon on the CCHS faculty. Their concerns were engendered by the developments at the teaching hospital in Birmingham, where the new teaching hospital effectively closed its doors to all of the qualified surgeons in the area. Eventually, only the salaried surgeons on the medical school faculty had hospital privileges. Although this concern was not unique to the surgeons, they are the only specialists whose workplace was confined to the hospital.

Willard met with the local surgeons with this in mind and proposed that they organize a teaching surgical service to serve the college, which would make the hiring of a full-time surgeon for the faculty unnecessary. Dr. William Shamblin, who was well respected and academically oriented, volunteered to organize the surgeons of the town into what would become an excellent and popular teaching program. Shamblin served as chair of the new surgical department and was soon joined by Mrs. Nickole L. Moore as the administrative assistant in the department, who went on to serve more than twenty-five years in this capacity.

The next professional to join the group was Dr. Douglas Scutchfield, who graduated from the University of Kentucky Medical Center in 1966.

Willard asked him to join the program as first head of the Department of Family and Community Medicine, and he went on to hold various other positions over the years, including associate dean of academic affairs for the college.

By the end of 1974, other individuals had joined the fledgling program. Dr. Robert Pieroni, with a medical degree from the Pennsylvania State University and a recently completed residency in Massachusetts, joined the staff as the second internist. Certified in both family medicine and internal medicine, Pieroni would prove to be a valuable addition to the teaching efforts of the college.

At the same time Dr. James Gascoigne and Dr. Russell Anderson came aboard as family practitioners. Anderson, who received his medical degree from the University of Kentucky and completed a residency at Mercy Medical Center in Ohio, was to spend almost twenty years with the college. He served as longtime head of the family medicine department and director of the residency program for several years as well. He had been in private practice for several years before joining Willard's faculty. "[I was] motivated by idealism about a better way of teaching medicine, a commitment to delivering care to rural areas and willing to fight status quo academic medicine." He was a strong addition to the college's efforts in family medicine.

Willard then hired Dr. Roland Ficken, with a Ph.D. in medical sociology, who had experience in the medical school at the University of Kentucky. Ficken agreed to develop the behavioral science department for the college, a significant discipline in Willard's growing program. With Ficken and the various support personnel who rounded out the program, Willard now had the makings of a bona fide medical education program.

The Medical Student Question

Although the medical education program was designed to train medical students and have a residency in family practice, there was some early controversy surrounding the question of whether medical students would be part of the Tuscaloosa campus. A few vocal members of the hospital's medical staff felt that having medical students involved with patients in the hospital would impair the efficiency of patient care, while having family practice residents would do the opposite. The original architects of the program had built it on the premise that exposure to family medicine, preferably during medical school, would encourage more young people to choose careers in this field. Thus, the college would serve as a campus devoted to the clinical portion of the medical school. Third- and fourth-year students could receive that portion of their education—including a curriculum with healthy doses of family medicine, community medicine, and behavioral science—in Tuscaloosa.

Although the CCHS faculty was very thin and the curriculum had not yet been fully developed, the first wave of students was sent to Tuscaloosa in October 1973 at the request of the administrators in Birmingham, who were facing a serious problem with overcrowding. The school's building program had fallen seriously behind, and with the increase in class sizes that had been recently implemented, UAB lacked the facilities to accommodate their third-year class. Both Huntsville and Tuscaloosa were asked to help with teaching for a three-month period.

Because the program was not fully developed, questions were raised about how to best accommodate the incoming students. Willard elected to assign the students to general practitioners in the area and to the embryonic family practice clinic for their one-month electives. Fortunately, several area physicians came forward to teach. Enthusiasm for medical education was high in the community as nearly thirty years had elapsed since the university had medical students. Some members of the medical community in particular looked forward to cultivating students' intellectual development and shaping the values and experiences of those who would one day be their professional peers.

Within a short time, however, the realities of teaching became obvious. Attitudes quickly changed as the students took their places in the physicians' busy offices. The doctors who had volunteered to teach, many without any previous teaching experience, soon discovered that the students seriously hampered their productivity: the time associated with teaching students while treating patients was considerable. Taking patient histories, examining patients, making diagnoses and therapeutic decisions, and running a practice with several inexperienced and often young students in tow was no easy task. Soon many doctors were complaining about the burden that teaching placed on them; few indicated they would ever do it again.

This experience, according to Willard, eventually created some opposition to sponsoring a medical student program in Tuscaloosa.[47] The town physicians could easily visualize the presence of family practice residents and the help they could provide. But medical students were an entirely different matter: the doctors viewed inexperienced medical students as being in the way. Even some faculty in the Department of Family Practice voiced opposition to the medical student program.

This manner of thinking concerned Willard greatly. Although the medical student education was not his top priority at that point, he did reflect that the lack of medical students would seriously "undermine" the program.[48] In order to address this program, a weekend retreat was planned in Birmingham. Here Willard presented his plans for the college and his aspirations for it, which included a medical student program. Discussions were held and by Sunday, the group voted to support a medical student program.

The next step then was convincing the staff at DCH. Although they had warmly welcomed the first installment of medical students, they too had soured on the idea of hosting medical students at the hospital. Willard met with the medical staff shortly after the retreat and discussed his plans for the college, and again the staff voted to support the program. Thus was the door opened for the education of medical students in Tuscaloosa. One can imagine the relief that Willard felt.

Building Program Takes Root

Another major undertaking that Mathews and Willard began in 1972–73 was the construction of physical facilities for the new program. State Senator Shelby had helped to secure $4 million for capital construction at both the Tuscaloosa and Huntsville campuses, and Mathews was anxious to get the building program up and running. Extensive planning began as soon as Willard arrived on campus.

The temporary administrative offices of the evolving medical education program were housed in the large, four-story Student Health Services building on University Boulevard. Although the new program initially consisted of only a few staff members, it was clear that more space would be needed as faculty members were recruited. Of course, the space requirements of the new medical education program were understandably vague because so much of the program was still undefined. But a few key elements were already recognized as being vital to a successful program, and Willard and Mathews got right to the job of planning facilities.

One of the well-recognized and much needed elements of the program was a clinical base for the new school, and DCH had agreed to serve in this capacity. Originally designed as a community hospital, DCH did not contain the educational space that would be needed for medical students and residents. Administrators at DCH and UA envisioned an educational tower that would contain teaching spaces, spaces for faculty development, and on-call rooms for residents. Also envisioned was space for a new health sciences library. The library developed by the college was currently located in the main library on the campus quadrangle, central to the campus, but geographically separate from the clinical activities it was designed to support. The proposed education tower would provide handsome new space for the library as well as ready access by students, residents, and the hospital medical staff and nurses. At that time the resources of the library—about 3,500 bound volumes—were growing under the stewardship of Barbara Doughty, who served as one of the first reference librarians for the Health Sciences Library, a position she held for twenty-one years.

Before the education tower could be developed, however, numerous issues had to be resolved. Arrangements had to be worked out that dealt with leasing the land from the hospital, paying for utilities, janitorial services, and so on. Another pressing issue related to a definition of how the tower would operate: nervous DCH administrators wanted no patient care activities to take place in the tower, as they could be viewed as competing with hospital activities. This stipulation was agreed upon and the logistical details were worked out; construction began in 1977.

Perhaps the most important aspect of the program was an outpatient clinic, which would allow for clinical teaching and would provide the headquarters for the clinical operations of the college. Such a facility was an integral part of the planned family practice residency, and as such was a requirement for operating an accredited program for the training of family physicians. Residents, medical students, and other allied health professionals would work and learn there under the supervision of specialists in family medicine, pediatrics, internal medicine, surgery, obstetrics and gynecology, and psychiatry. Moore, as assistant dean for administration, led the planning for this effort. Ground breaking occurred on September 27, 1973. The 30,000-square-foot facility, called the Family Practice Clinic (later to be known as Capstone Medical Center), was built on University Boulevard, directly across the street from DCH on university-owned property. Opened in 1975, the multispecialty clinic offered a unique approach to the training of family practice physicians.

The clinic was designed so that the family practice residents, divided into four teams, would have a clinical home base, a physician's office. Each team, consisting of first-, second- and third-year residents, would see their patients for the duration of their training. Only the faculty would rotate periodically so that the residents could experience various approaches to patient care. Each resident was required to develop a panel of patients for whom he or she provided continuing care—a major element of family practice.

The faculty in the other major specialties had their own suites, including internal medicine, pediatrics, psychiatry, and obstetrics and gynecology. As the faculty developed an interest in occupational medicine, a suite was added for that subspecialty as well. The residents would also rotate through these suites, but teaching here was more directed at the medical students.

Administrative space was also a necessity, and for sentimental reasons, a suggestion was made that Nott Hall be renovated (the facility was by this time in a state of disrepair) and enlarged to house the new college. Renovations began in 1974 and were paid for with the $4 million appropriated by the Legislature.

Although the administrators of the new program got off to a running start with the building efforts, there was an interim period when space was not yet available. Thus in October of 1973, CCHS rented space in the former offices of Dr. E. C. Brock near the hospital to serve as a temporary ambulatory clinic. Here, the first few physicians on the staff started to see patients. "Dr. Willard was anxious to appear 'more medical' by starting to see patients," said Packard, who was on the staff at the time, noting that he was the only internist on the faculty and the program did not yet have residents. This temporary space was crowded and inefficient in many ways, but it served its purpose until the Family Practice Center opened for business in 1975.

Changes in Governance

While the administrators in Tuscaloosa were rapidly building the medical education program, administrators at UAB were also busy with the program there, which was undergoing tremendous changes of its own in the early 1970s. Many were completely independent of the new programs in Tuscaloosa and Huntsville, but would have an ultimate impact on the medical education programs throughout the state. One was UAB's recent adoption of a new curriculum, which allowed for graduation from medical school in as few as three years (instead of the traditional four). The justification given for this shorter curriculum, which was being adopted in several U.S. medical schools, was that it could provide the same training at lower cost in time and money and would get young doctors out of school one year earlier, thus giving them an extra year to serve communities. For the state of Alabama, this was another way to address the growing physician shortage.

At the same time, UASOM was growing: the school had gone from accepting eighty students to 125 students per class, a substantial difference requiring a major commitment of additional resources. Of the major changes taking place in the system, only this one would stand the test of time.

At the same time the university system was being criticized on several fronts. With state funds low and money being appropriated to Tuscaloosa, Huntsville, and Mobile for medical education, there was pressure on the university's board of trustees. Citizens and politicians alike voiced concerns about the duplication of efforts in the state, the need for coordination of all of the various medical education programs, and a fear that the state would try to develop four complete medical schools (including two news ones at Tuscaloosa and Huntsville).

In response a group from UAB, chaired by Dr. S. Richardson Hill, held a series of meetings during the summer of 1972 with the goal of developing a workable system of governance for medical education in the University of Alabama system. In attendance were Dr. Clifton Meador, dean of UASOM; Dr. Bud Grulee, a representative from the UAH, which had not yet appointed a dean; Dean Robert Bucher of the University of South Alabama; and Willard of the Tuscaloosa campus. The meetings, which were later described by Willard as both cordial and productive, were intended to coordinate a medical education program between the three campuses, plus the University of South Alabama, with an eye toward taking "full advantage of all of Alabama's current assets in medical education."

The resulting report prepared by Hill laid out a loosely formulated system of governance for the medical system, with particular emphasis on the evolving new programs in Tuscaloosa and Huntsville. The report recognized the changes taking place in the system and the role that the two branch campuses might play in terms of strengthening medical education in Alabama: certainly, opportunities for clinical clerkships, electives, and residency programs could be greatly expanded with the use of these additional faculties, community hospitals, and other resources. Hill wrote that each institution should have full control over its own budget, but that a coordination of budgets from the three campuses was necessary before submission to the appropriate state agency. Accreditation, the report went on to explain, would be obtained through UAB's medical school, with the intent that at some later date, "independent accreditation for the house-staff program could be sought."

Hill's work was then used as the basis for the completed document, which was prepared by Judge Daniel T. McCall, Jr., a member of the board of trustees and justice of the State Supreme Court. Judge McCall, who was the son of the last dean of the medical school in Mobile before it was moved to Tuscaloosa in 1920 and hence had a personal interest in medical education in Alabama, had been asked to head up a committee to study the subject of how to best govern the medical education programs in the state. In addition to Hill's work, the committee relied on the advice of Dr. Charles "Mickey" LeMaistre, an alumnus of UA and the chancellor of the University of Texas medical school system, who counseled the board about the organization of medical education at the University of Texas and its relation to the total system. With his input and the report written by Hill, McCall and his Special Committee of the Board for System Medical Programs prepared a final report, which came to be known as the McCall report and was the governing document for the three-campus medical education system.

Although the McCall report established a degree of autonomy for each campus, it directed that Hill would supervise the UAB medical program and all of the campuses. Willard, Mathews, and the staff at DCH took exception to the fact that Birmingham would supervise the activities in Tuscaloosa. According to Willard, this was when the first strain in the relationship with Birmingham occurred. Willard had been hired by Mathews and his loyalty lay with him, not the administration in Birmingham. This conflict between the two schools resulted in a number of complaints made to both Birmingham and the university's board of trustees. Later, a meeting was held between Hill and Willard, at which Willard expressed his concerns that Birmingham would try to "control" Tuscaloosa. However, nothing came from these attempts at changing the governance structure between the schools, and the McCall report was never revised to satisfy Willard. The document, however, would be revisited repeatedly over the next two decades, as the concerns over governance issues were resolved.

About this time another key change was made to the medical school structure with the addition of a new dean of the University of Alabama School of Medicine, Dr. James A. Pittman, Jr., who replaced Meador, dean since 1968. A native of Florida with a medical degree from Harvard University, Pittman completed residencies at both Massachusetts General Hospital and UAB. He then went on to the National Cancer Institute in Bethesda, Maryland, for another period of study, before returning to the Department of Medicine in Birmingham in 1956 as chief resident under Dr. Tinsley Harrison. Following his residency he was asked to join the faculty. With research interests in endocrinology and nuclear medicine, he taught for many years and assumed additional administrative responsibilities over the years, including director of the Division of Endocrinology. Long involved with the Veterans Administration, Pittman left UAB in 1971 for a brief stint as chief medical director for Research and Education in Medicine for the Veterans Administration in Washington, D.C. He returned to Alabama in 1973 when he accepted the post of dean of the medical school under Dr. S. Richardson Hill, vice president for Health Affairs. Pittman would serve the medical school in this capacity for nineteen years; over this time he would have a great deal of influence over the medical education programs in Tuscaloosa.

The Education Process Begins

The first full-time students to enter the program at CCHS arrived in early 1974; they only numbered three. They had been recruited from two-year medical schools in North Dakota and Nevada. And like all of the medical students who came to CCHS during its fledgling years, they joined an untried program with no reputation or track record for the last two years of medical school. Coming to Tuscaloosa during this time must have required an act of faith. It was truly a brand-new venture and it offered a new and more personalized clinical medical education.

The Tuscaloosa campus of UASOM provided the full spectrum of clinical education in medicine. Like many of the branch campuses in the United States, it prepared medical graduates to go into a specialty or sub-specialty of their choice. Graduates are legally undifferentiated at the time they receive their medical degree. Thus, in spite of the emphasis on family practice in Tuscaloosa, the program was shaped to provide the full complement of third- and fourth-year medical courses of study. The medical student curriculum in Tuscaloosa was compatible with that offered in Birmingham and consisted of three months in internal medicine, pediatrics, and surgery; two months of obstetrics/gynecology, and one month of psychiatry. In addition, students were given one month of family medicine instead of a required fourth-year course in internal medicine. Emphasis was also placed on community medicine and behavioral science and a two-month elective in these areas was included. Community physician preceptors have been essential to this program from the beginning (Appendix C).

Responsibility for matters related to the medical students fell to Packard, as associate dean for Clinical Affairs. His office was structured to serve medical students on the Tuscaloosa campus, helping them to function as effectively as possible while achieving their educational goals. The main functions of this office included orientation of new students, career counseling, monitoring of student performance, administration of the National Board Examinations, maintenance of student records, and co-ordination of the National Intern and Resident Matching program.

The office handled other, unofficial duties as well. "I figured my job was to take all the minutiae out of the students' lives and let them learn. I took care of all the rotation scheduling, enrollment, and any kind of dealing they might have with the university. That was my job and I said, 'You just learn to be a good doctor,'" said Mary Leta Taylor, who served as the staff assistant in the office of medical student affairs, a position she held from 1973 to 1991. Taylor, who described working with the CCHS medical students as "a joy" in her life, described the first medical students who came through the Tuscaloosa program. "Most of the students went into medicine because they wanted to help people, and I don't think that's changed. [I always found them to be] happy with who they are and what they are doing. I think that is attributable to coming to this campus where their role models were not off in a lab somewhere, but were hard-working people who were taking good care of patients and not off writing a book somewhere, making money or doing something else. I think they were well aware that all of the teaching physicians could make a lot more money if they were in private practice, but they were dedicated to teaching," she said.

Teaching the first groups of students started slowly for several reasons. The college had only a small faculty on which to draw and a handful of volunteer physicians in the community. Most of these were inexperienced teachers working from a curriculum that was still evolving. Likewise, faculty turnover in these early years was high and competing priorities of patient care, development of research programs, service, and teaching proved to be problematic. However, the CCHS medical education program did offer one key advantage and that was its small size, which made access to physicians easier. The CCHS program offered teaching by the attending physicians, not residents, and as such, students were exposed to more day-to-day patient care activities than was possible in much larger medical school settings (although the residents' responsibilities to supervise and teach students were established later).

Dr. Frank Dozier, now a private practitioner with his wife, Dr. Daveta Dozier, in Thomasville, Alabama, was in one of the early medical student classes at CCHS. In an interview he noted that many students opted to go to Tuscaloosa because it offered more opportunities for close contact with the faculty and the patients. "I felt like I wanted to go into family practice," he recalled, "and I wanted to know what the family practitioners and the residency program were like. And also I had heard that [the students in] the Tuscaloosa program had more hands-on experience. It had as much academics but more one-on-one with the faculty, especially in the surgery program. I figured as a student I probably wouldn't be able to do as much in Birmingham as I would if I went to Tuscaloosa."

Tuscaloosa did turn out to be an exceptional learning experience, he went on to say. "In talking to other students in Birmingham, they couldn't believe some of the things we were being involved in as medical students, and that continued until I completed the residency program." He remembered being encouraged to do procedures in pediatrics, surgery, and even the high-risk nursery, experiences that would enrich his education.

From the inception of the medical student program at CCHS, surgery would stand out as one of the most popular rotations in the program. Shamblin and several area doctors, all part-time faculty for CCHS, soon became recognized as excellent teachers, providing opportunities to get close to and even assist with surgical procedures. With no surgical residents or fellows, the medical students could assist in meaningful ways before, during, and after the surgical procedures. Soon many students from Birmingham, even if they did not opt to attend CCHS, would come to Tuscaloosa for the valuable experience in surgery; over the years, more than 140 Birmingham-based students have elected to take their third-year surgical rotations in Tuscaloosa, where they joined, for that rotation, the full-time students at CCHS.

Teaching in the surgical department benefited greatly from the addition of Dr. Joe Burleson, a retired orthopedic surgeon from Asheville, North Carolina, who joined CCHS in 1975 and helped organize the surgical program, taught students and residents, and eventually operated an orthopedic clinic in the Family Practice Center.

The appeal of the surgical rotation was due in part to the efforts that Shamblin made in preparation for his role as chair. He visited with the chief of surgery in Birmingham, Dr. John Kirklin, whom he had known during his own surgical residency at the Mayo Clinic. Shamblin became familiar with the structure and goals of the Birmingham program and modeled the Tuscaloosa program accordingly. In an interview, Shamblin reflected that ties were established with the surgical departments in Birmingham and then in Huntsville "so that we would have a three-campus system in the Department of Surgery that was more cohesive than separate."

"It turned out to be a good experience for all of us," he said.

As one of the primary care specialties, pediatrics also proved to be a popular and successful teaching service from its inception. Department chairman Hefelfinger sought the advice and support of colleagues in Birmingham, including the chairman of the pediatrics department, Dr. John Benton. A strong relationship was developed between the two departments, as a result, which led to frequent consultations with pediatric subspecialists in Birmingham and ultimately the establishment of subspecialty clinics at the Family Practice Clinic staffed by Birmingham faculty members.

Teaching in the Department of Family and Community Medicine was also strong from the start. Headed by Dr. Scutchfield, the department was primarily responsible for the residency program. However, the department's faculty developed and supervised the rural preceptor experience for medical students.

At the same time that the first medical students arrived on the UA campus, CCHS began to welcome its first residents. These newly graduated physicians signed on for a three-year training program in family practice. It was one of 140 such programs in the country in a rapidly growing and changing field. From the beginning of the residency it was obvious that the overall structure of the program would provide an excellent learning environment for the doctors in training. One benefit of the program was that it was the only residency program in the hospital; no other residencies competed for patients or faculty teaching time. The full-time faculty represented the core curricular areas of family medicine and many excellent and enthusiastic volunteer faculty rounded out the experience. Furthermore, the presence of third- and fourth-year medical students in a well-established college town added to the academic environment.

The January 1974 arrival of Dr. Marc Armstrong as the new program's first resident signaled the launching of the residency. A graduate of Tulane, Armstrong, who would later play a major role in the college as a member of the faculty, described feeling like he was "the center of the universe" as the first resident.

Within several months, others joined the residency. In July, Dr. Michael McBrearty joined the program, having transferred from the University of Oklahoma family practice residency. McBrearty had previously done a student rotation with Dr. Rutland in Fayette. It was about this time that Rutland would take on a new role in the residency program himself, agreeing to serve as its acting director after Hubbard left to return to Florida.

In November 1974, two other residents joined the program, Dr. Tim Simmons, who transferred from the St. Margaret's program in Pittsburgh, Pennsylvania, and Dr. Larry Sullivan, a graduate of UASOM.

From the very beginning of the family practice residency, the quality of the people who entered the program was high and happily recognized as such. Dianne Kerr, a nurse at the Capstone Medical Center for more than twenty-five years, noted that it was the quality of those early residents that "sparked" her interest in working for the clinic. "You know I have had the privilege of working with the most wonderful human beings and physicians in the whole world, and I am very, very thankful," she said in an interview.

Such was the excellence of the program from its very early days. In the years to follow, it would continue to fill out as more residents and students opted to pursue their education at CCHS.

4
Growing Pains

By the mid-1970s much of the hard, initial work of developing a basic structure for the school had been completed: the family practice residency program was approved and under way, a clinical program for undergraduate medical students had been formed, and several excellent faculty and administrators had been hired. The dean and his new staff had worked extremely hard and well, and the program was beginning to take shape.

An Evolving Program

By 1975 CCHS had undergone a great deal of growth and development. It was a time for building, but also for change. In the university administration, modifications were under way in response to the temporary departure of President Mathews for Washington, D.C., where he was asked to serve as the secretary of the U.S. Department of Health, Education and Welfare under President Gerald Ford. During his absence, Professor Richard Thigpen served as acting chief executive officer of the university.

The year would be filled with accomplishment, including most notably the opening of the new Family Practice Center on University Boulevard, the base of the college's clinical program. In June the staff moved into the new 30,000 square-foot facility with great fanfare. The grand opening of the facility in August was attended by numerous dignitaries, including Lady Bird Johnson, wife of former President Lyndon Johnson. The local newspaper extolled the opening of the new facility, which, it reported, was not only "a great addition to the services offered by the state's comprehensive university here, but . . . a challenging new asset for Tuscaloosa."[49]

Progress was also being made on the new education tower at DCH.

While construction on the tower would not begin until 1977, planning efforts, including negotiations with the hospital, were well underway. The administration hoped that the facility would be available to serve the residents and faculty working at the hospital by 1977 or 1978.

The middle of the decade also brought the establishment of a critical bond between CCHS and the Veterans Administration Hospital, an affiliation that would benefit both organizations. Nationally, the VA system serves not only as a source of medical care for veterans, but also provides an important vehicle for medical education. In fact, by 1975, more than half of all U.S. medical students received at least some of their medical training in VA facilities.[50] In 1972 the VA was providing grant money to medical schools that had affiliations with the VA: the long-term goal was to improve the quality of patient care at veterans' facilities by involving medical school faculty members, residents, and students in patient care. In 1975 Willard, with help from administrators in Birmingham, including the dean of UASOM, Pittman, received a grant for more than $7 million over seven years. The funds would be used to assist with operating costs and various building projects, such as the renovation of the fourth floor of the Student Health Center, which served as office space for CCHS faculty for many years.

The second component of the relationship between the VA and the college involved the veterans hospital located in Tuscaloosa, one of four in the state. The 700-bed psychiatric hospital, located a few miles from the university campus, provides health care services to eligible veterans in the region. The college administration realized that the center could serve as a valuable resource for teaching medical students and residents. The program became reality in 1977 with the signing of an affiliation agreement between the two organizations. For many years this would serve as an important training ground for family practice residents and medical students in the diagnosis and management of psychiatric disorders. One benefit was the fifty-bed acute medical ward, where patients with serious medical problems could receive long-term treatment without concerns about early discharge for financial reasons. Here students and residents participated in the care of patients under the supervision of Dr. Patrick McCue, longtime director of Medical Education at the VA and a gifted teacher.

On a personal level, 1975 marked an important achievement for Willard, who was awarded the AMA's prestigious Distinguished Service

Award, its highest honor. This award was given in recognition of his service to the field of medical education, including the development of the guidelines for the formal specialty of family practice.

Building the Residency

The family practice residency program at CCHS was also being strengthened during this time. In January 1975 three new first-year residents joined the program and by July, twelve more were added. This was the first time that a full class of residents had joined the program. As the number of residents grew, the need for additional structure became obvious. The residents were organized into four teams, each composed of first-, second-, and third-year residents. Each team shared night call, emergencies, and patients for the duration of the program.

In 1976 Dr. William deShazo was recruited to a new role as director of the residency program, and the first class he recruited would be a memorable one. In this class were the first African-Americans to join the residency: Dr. Herb Stone, a Georgia native who had recently earned his medical degree from Emory, and Dr. Sandral Hullett, a native of Alabama and a recent graduate of the Medical College of Pennsylvania. Hullett was also the first female resident in the program. This was a major step for the Tuscaloosa program, only thirteen years after George Wallace's infamous stand at the schoolhouse door. Although deShazo was criticized by some for hiring the first blacks to the program, he had hired two highly qualified residents, chosen because they were such strong candidates, not because of their race.

After their arrival, deShazo worked hard to ensure that Stone and Hullett were made to feel comfortable. "Dr. deShazo was concerned about how I was going to feel if a person didn't want to see me if I was black," explained Hullett in a recent interview. "I felt confident about who I was with my skills, I didn't have much trouble relating to people who, when you walk in, they say, 'I'm here to see the doctor.' I would say, 'I'm it.' And then usually they would calm down and they felt better."

A key contributor to her comfort level was the support she received from her team of residents, a group she described as very close-knit. "They [her fellow residents] all sat down and they said to me, 'You are a member of this team and so if a patient can't see you, they can't see anybody in the group.' And that was so very important to me," she said, "because they gave me the support I needed to feel comfortable doing things." Hullett also spoke of the pressure associated with being the first female in the residency and one of the first blacks.

"At first, I had a level of confidence, you know, I felt good, but I was also uncomfortable too, sometimes more uncomfortable than the people I was seeing. I wanted to do good, I didn't want to make any mistakes, I felt sort of in a fishbowl situation because I didn't want to make a mistake," she said.

Her determination to "do good" would later be exemplified in her career. After graduating from the residency, Hullett went on to have a successful career as a rural practitioner. She has received several honors, including induction into the Alabama Academy of Honor and the National Institute of Medicine, a unit of the National Academy of Sciences. She was named Rural Doctor of the Year by the National Rural Health Association in 1988. Hullett would also play a key role in the oversight of the University of Alabama System during her twelve years on the board of trustees.

According to deShazo, witnessing such success stories was a highlight of his career. "The most rewarding thing is to have been able to help recruit these residents and follow them through the years and see what they have done with their lives. Look at the people that have been president of the Alabama Academy of Family Practice of this state who are graduates [of the residency]. Look at the president of the academy in Louisiana. Look at where these people have stayed, they have gone to small towns and stayed. That has been the most pleasant and rewarding part," he said (Appendix E). The joy deShazo took in the success of others was one of the qualities that had made him such an outstanding choice to head the residency program. At the residents' request, the faculty in Family Medicine established the William F. deShazo, Jr., Award, to be presented each year to the outstanding resident in family medicine at the completion of the three-year program.

CCHS Reaches Out

By the middle of the decade the college also had undertaken several outreach programs—a vital element of Willard's new models of patient care in Alabama. Programs that were under way at that time included the initiation of a continuing medical education program for physicians in the area, service by the faculty at a number of community health clinics, the establishment of a primary care clinic in rural West Blocton, Alabama, and the organization of a family practice residency program in Selma-Dallas County, Alabama, with Dr. Donald Overstreet serving as director.

One of the most significant outreach efforts of the time was the establishment of a clinic for minorities in the western section of Tuscaloosa, later to be called the Maude L. Whatley Health Center. The effort was the brainchild of a group of CCHS medical students who were concerned about the noticeable lack of health care available to minorities in the city. They took the initiative to organize a weekly clinic at a temporary location off of Greensboro Avenue in Tuscaloosa and enlisted the assistance of residents, nursing students, and faculty to join in the effort. Chairman of the Department of Behavioral Sciences Dr. Roland Ficken took a leading role in supporting the effort and with the help of Dr. Suzanne Medgyesi-Mitshang, executive assistant to the dean, soon prepared a grant application for submission to the U.S. Department of Health, Education and Welfare (HEW). When the grant was approved, funding amounted to almost $500,000, which enabled the clinic to move from a temporary location on Herman Avenue to a larger, permanent facility on Martin Luther King, Jr. Blvd. Today the clinic continues as a designated federal community health center serving more than 11,000 people each year.

During the late 1970s CCHS also embarked on several collaborative projects with other units of the University. Willard was working to reestablish a nursing education program in Tuscaloosa. The former school of nursing was moved to the Birmingham campus in 1966, to be associated with the university teaching hospital. After much work this program received funding by the State Legislature in 1976, and a new College of Nursing was formed. Strong ties between the two schools were established, and CCHS faculty had agreed to teach several behavioral science courses to nursing students and provide a teaching setting at the new Family Practice Center.

Over the years the clinic would serve a distinctive role on campus as a key learning center for students from many UA programs and even students from other local colleges, including Shelton State Community College in Tuscaloosa. Margaret Garner, a nutritionist and member of the Department of Family Medicine for more than twenty-three years, explained the value that the center has had in teaching students at every level about different aspects of health care.

"Over the years this center has provided a key learning laboratory experience for students in psychology, social work, dietetics, nursing, speech and language pathology, occupational therapy, physical therapy, and health care management. This has been an incredible resource to the university community, more than we have publicized ourselves to be, and I'm very, very proud of that," she said.

Garner, who has served for many years on the UA Faculty Senate, helped forge the bonds with these other programs, establishing a critical link between CCHS and the other colleges on campus. As such she spent a great deal of time communicating with UA faculty about the goals and missions of the College, including the service component.

During the mid-1970s a tie was formed with the College of Commerce and Business Administration to sponsor an undergraduate program in health care management. The program, which had more than 100 students enrolled by 1976, involved coursework in a variety of health care–related areas taught by the CCHS faculty or clinic managers, dealing with the nonclinical aspects of health care delivery.

Although these activities fulfilled a need on campus and in the community, they were viewed by administrators in Birmingham as peripheral to the basic mission of teaching medical students and residents. Dean Pittman expressed his expectation that the CCHS faculty would focus on this basic mission, especially in view of the fact that questions still lingered about the quality of medical education on the Tuscaloosa campus.

Two Different Philosophies

Differences in the philosophies between the two organizations and their leaders drove a wedge between CCHS and UASOM. Willard and Pittman believed in two contrasting elements in medical education. These were not mutually exclusive, one being an emphasis on the patient and the disease, the other being an emphasis on patient and the family, psychosocial relationships, and the community. The differences could have been compromised, but beneath these were yet more basic concerns. Pittman believed that Willard's philosophy and experience were too centered in public health and preventive medicine. Indeed, Willard and

Mathews embraced the opportunity to develop integrative programs that would fit with Mathews' convictions regarding the role of "community" and Willard's conviction that attention to this important element of health care would improve the quality, availability, and utilization of health care services in Alabama.

In Birmingham Dean Pittman thought differently. Here, the thrust was not in solving the broad general health problems of the Alabama populace, but in the more prevalent and exciting biomedical research that could bring new insight into the causes of disease and then to specific methods of cure. Indeed, success with this approach has brought grateful patients to the teaching hospital and distinction to the medical center in Birmingham—and to Alabama. "Research," he wrote in a 1995 essay for the *American Journal of Medical Sciences,* "is the most reforming of all health care strategies."[51]

But many in medicine have pointed out the flaws inherent in this approach. Dr. Gayle Stephens, former dean of the School of Primary Care at the UAH, wrote that the so-called reductionist approach had led to a preoccupation with a "knowledge of parts," resulting in a fragmented view of the human body. "This view has had a very salutary effect in certain categories of diseases," he wrote, "but it has been fruitless in maladies that have psychological, social or cultural determinants."[52]

Many worried about the lack of attention being paid to maintaining good health in the general population. It appeared that many of the determinants of good health were being neglected as the country raced ahead in research.[53] Willard perceived that public health was being neglected in this respect, and that this was reflected in the medical education methods of the day.

Such was the reality of the situation and at least part of the problem between the two schools. Pittman, for his part, would refer publicly to the "divergence" of the Tuscaloosa program from what he viewed as the school's only proper goal: medical education. Dr. Harry Knopke, who served as the associate dean of Academic Affairs for eight years, noted that the main problem between the two campuses was a distinctly different philosophy. He noted that Mathews saw the community as a whole. "He saw the university as a land grant institution and he believed you should take parts of the university out to the community. His worldview coincided perfectly with Willard's."

However, their view did not coincide with that of the many of the administrators in Birmingham, and this lack of philosophical agreement led to years of strained relations within the medical school.

Accreditation Problems

But the imperfect relationship between the two schools was not the only problem facing Dean Willard in 1975, for this year was the first Liaison Committee on Medical Education (LCME) review of the branch campuses in Tuscaloosa and Huntsville. And for CCHS, the results of the review of the undergraduate medical education program represented a major stumbling block in the development of the UA program.

The LCME is an international accrediting organization established in 1942 as a cooperative effort between AAMC and the Council on Medical Education and Hospitals of the AMA. In 1968 the LCME was recognized by the U.S. government as being the official organization for accreditation of medical schools. As such, the LCME establishes criteria for the educational, financial, and physical status for all medical schools. Accreditation is critical for the survival of a medical school since most state licensing boards require applicants to graduate from accredited institutions in order to be eligible for licensure.

New schools or major changes made to existing programs are normally surveyed several times during their first few years. Such programs are typically accredited provisionally. Established medical schools are surveyed at regular intervals, typically every eight years. The criteria used to accredit U.S. medical schools were to be found in important documents published by the LCME: "The Functions and Structure of a Medical School" and "Special Criteria for Programs in Basic Medical Sciences." In 1975, just as UASOM prepared for their accreditation review, a third document was being prepared by the LCME, this one dealing specifically with the issues associated with branch campuses such as Tuscaloosa and Huntsville. Unsure of how to assess the quality of the relatively large number of off-campus programs being instituted around the country at satellite sites, the LCME drew up "Supplemental Guidelines for Branch Campuses" and circulated them for comment in 1975. It was in this environment, with a growing national concern about the quality of off-campus branches, that UASOM would undergo its review.

The major accreditation review that took place in September 1975 involved a thorough examination of the established medical school in Birmingham and the branch campuses in Tuscaloosa and Huntsville. The LCME review process is long and complex and involves a self-study by the organization to be reviewed, followed by a site visit by LCME representatives. The site visit team gives a preliminary report to the dean of the medical school and the president of the university. A formal report stating the outcome of the review is sent from the LCME in the weeks or months to follow.

In preparation for the 1975 review, the staff and faculty at Tuscaloosa made its preparations. Willard appointed Ficken to take the lead on the review and be involved with the logistics of the visit. The intensive, three-day site visit was conducted by a group of six reviewers, who visited with representatives and students at Tuscaloosa, Birmingham, and Huntsville. In Tuscaloosa, the group met with members of the faculty and staff, several residents, representatives of DCH, and some local physicians.

At the end of the visit, as is customary, the review team met with the leadership, including Dean Pittman and Vice President Hill. They also spent a short amount of time with the deans in Tuscaloosa and Huntsville pointing out areas for improvement. After their visit the review team wrote a summary of its observations, which was transmitted to the school as an unofficial report. The primary issues of concern observed by the review team involved issues of governance as spelled out in the draft supplemental guidelines. Everyone at the three schools was certain that the team would make recommendations for changes and perhaps schedule a return visit a bit early to see what progress had been made.

But nothing in the visit or the follow-up report prepared the school for the full brunt of the decision handed down by the LCME in April 1976. In its official notification to the university, the LCME was critical of the overall program, limiting the accreditation to three years. This was the first time since the medical school in Birmingham had been founded in 1945 that such a restriction had been put on the school. Problems associated with governance were emphasized by the group, but they were also extremely critical of the program at CCHS. They stipulated that the Tuscaloosa program would be limited to only twelve medical students in each class and that these students must first complete six months of clinical work in Birmingham before transferring to this campus.

Both Willard and his faculty were disappointed by the results of the review. "This came as a great surprise to us because we did not feel that our program was deficient in any serious way and we also felt we were doing as good a job as Huntsville was doing," wrote Willard.[54]

"Needless to say, we were extremely disappointed," recalled Ficken in an interview. "But we were neophytes, all of us except Dr. Willard, and it showed in our approach to the visit." Ficken also added that Huntsville did a much better job of "selling" their program.

Correspondence at this time reflects the frustration of the faculty. Willard in particular was chagrined by the results of the review and the restrictions put on the system. In the area of governance, in particular, he saw the decree of the LCME as putting undue pressure on a system that was still very new. "Under the present organization of UASMEP, the dean of the School of Medicine at Birmingham is put in an impossible situation," he wrote in August 1976 in an internal document. "He is held accountable for the quality of the undergraduate medical education at the Tuscaloosa and Huntsville campuses. However, the decentralization of administrative authority within the university to the campus presidents, and in turn, to the dean of the College of Community Health Sciences at Tuscaloosa and the dean of the School of Primary Medical Care at Huntsville does not give him the authority to make changes when and where he and his faculty might think this is indicated." Willard expressed concern that the attempt by the LCME to centralize the authority and resources of the program would essentially cripple the two branch campus programs. He feared that the arrangement would lead to less effective relationships with local people and organizations because UAB representatives were not in a position to respond to local needs. And, Willard worried that the opportunities for innovation and initiative would be lost under such an arrangement. He believed that without any authority he and the dean in Huntsville would be completely ineffective, in a system that would be so cumbersome that it could not help but break down. Willard remained adamant—he never agreed to submit to Pittman's authority. His resignation in 1978 was due to this and to Mathews's departure to HEW. On Mathews's return, he had other fish to fry, and no longer supported Willard. They were bound to lose in any event.

The Fallout

The results of the LCME visit of 1975 were a major source of consternation for the administrators and faculty in Birmingham, and much was done in the following year to try to rectify the perceived weaknesses in the program. One of the major efforts initiated by the university board of trustees was to undertake a study to evaluate the programs in Birmingham, Huntsville, and Tuscaloosa. The board turned to a group of consultants led by Dr. William Stewart, then commissioner of the Louisiana Health and Human Resources Administration. Stewart was assisted by Dr. Christopher C. Fordham, III, dean of the School of Medicine at the University of North Carolina and Dr. Max Michael, Jr., assistant dean of the School of Medicine at the University of Florida and head of the branch campus in Jacksonville. The group spent five days in August 1976 scrutinizing the Alabama medical education program. The results of their visit were conveyed to vice president Hill in a document that became known as the Stewart report. In it the consultants recognized the many accomplishments made in the medical education program in the years since the McCall report was issued. However, they could not ignore the many governance issues plaguing the campus. "The School of Medicine faculty in Birmingham, with its administrative officers, is not unequivocally in charge of the entire education program," the report's authors wrote. Their primary recommendation was direct: abandon the clinical programs at both Tuscaloosa and Huntsville. The three consultants felt that developing the two programs "would be a mistake." Instead the group envisioned a completely different role for the two branch campuses and suggested they might be more useful converted into "area health education centers."

Such centers are part of a federally funded program designed to educate medical students, resident physicians, and other health care personnel in underserved or remote areas. Enacted in 1972, the intent of the program was to improve the geographic distribution of physicians, thus insuring the availability of essential health care services for 95 percent of all Americans. In Alabama, such a change would shift the focus toward a broad-based approach to health education for the rural areas of the state, but away from the more limited education of medical students. This proposal represented a radical change in course, one that was deemed unacceptable to many in the state who had been involved with the firm, expensive commitment that had been made to medical education in both Huntsville and Tuscaloosa.

The Stewart report resulted in a great deal of dialogue between the three campuses; strong disagreement was voiced about how best to proceed. Dr. Pittman, who was extremely concerned about the LCME view of the program, believed the best way to resolve the issues at hand was to accept the recommendation of the Stewart report and change the nature of the programs at Huntsville and Tuscaloosa. In this way funds for undergraduate medical education would be funneled through Birmingham while other programs, such as the allied health efforts, might be funded directly through each branch campus. In Huntsville Stephens wished to centralize the program and thus have closer ties to Birmingham. Willard preferred to keep the system as it was.

Others outside the Alabama system criticized the Stewart report. Dr. Andrew J. Rudnick, vice president and dean of faculties at the University of Houston, provided comments to Vice President Hill on the results of the review by Stewart and his colleagues. Rudnick disagreed strongly with the conclusions of the report and instead noted that the state of Alabama had made "real progress" in only five years on its medical education program and expressed his belief that the consultants had "seemingly ignored the rationale for so many qualified people (whether professional or lay) lending their support to those programs." In his letter to UAB, he also wrote in support of the "commendable goals set by Judge McCall and the Board of Trustees."

Hill, for his part, reserved judgment on the Stewart report and directed the deans of the three campuses to make a combined response to him about how to handle the recommendations made by the consultants. Numerous attempts to do this were made, including one in November 1976. In a sixteen-page memorandum to Hill from Pittman, each recommendation in the Stewart report was addressed in detail. But like other attempts to address the conflicting concerns of the group, the document only seemed to highlight further the differences between the three institutions and their respective deans. In the end, the deans agreed to "be guided by" the principles laid out in the report and to work toward repairing any deficiencies in the system. However, they also agreed not to implement them in detail.

The feelings about the report at UA may have best been summed up by Scutchfield, by then Associate Dean for CCHS, who wrote to Willard in a memo of his frustration with reviews of this sort. "It seems to me that during the past two years we have lived from crisis to crisis, from site visit to site visit. It seems to me that we need to have clear articulation as to what they expect out of CCHS in the next 5–10 years." It was a feeling of frustration shared by many.

The Next Test for the College

The years that followed were a time of tremendous change and challenge for the university system including CCHS. At every level, the impact of decreased funding could be felt. Federal dollars, so plentiful in the 1960s and early 1970s, were less available to educational institutions. The double-digit inflation, high unemployment, and reduced revenues plaguing the country were felt in Alabama, too. Furthermore, the recent proliferation of junior colleges and technical schools in the state had stretched the resources of the state and money was extremely tight. In 1978, and again in 1979, state budgets to the university were prorated, thus exacerbating many of the problems within the system.

Administrative changes were also taking place at this time. In late 1976 the board of trustees named Dr. Joseph F. Volker, former president of UAB and builder of the well-respected dental school there, as first chancellor of The University of Alabama System. In this capacity, Volker was asked to act as an advocate for the university presidents and to ensure coordination between the three campuses, a move that was intended to strengthen the administration of the system. Hill was promoted to president of UAB in February 1977 but was also to continue as director of UASMEP. These changes sharpened the administrative focus for the university system.

Other changes were afoot in Tuscaloosa. In January 1977 Mathews returned to UA to resume his presidency of the Tuscaloosa campus after spending seventeen months in Washington, D.C. Mathews returned to his former job, where he found a discontented university faculty frustrated by a lack of growth in academic programs and salaries, and was soon forced to retire.

At the same time, Willard continued to work hard to build the college that he envisioned in 1972. Recruiting for the college continued unabated, and some key personnel joined CCHS during this time. One of these was Dr. Harry Knopke, who joined the faculty as an assistant professor in behavioral science and director of the medical student program in 1977. With a Master of Science degree and doctorate in education from the

University of Wisconsin–Madison, Knopke—with his outstanding skills as an intermediary and mediator—would become a vital member of the college and the university community for many years.

Willard, Knopke said, represented the major reason that he decided to move to Alabama. "What he wanted to do in Alabama and in the South was very appealing," he said, "in fact, it was compelling." After several years on the faculty, Knopke assumed the position of associate dean for Academic Affairs in the college, a position that would utilize his strengths in administration.

Another key addition in 1977 was Dr. William W. Winternitz, who was asked by Willard to head the Department of Internal Medicine. A native of Connecticut, Winternitz was the son of two physicians and had an impressive medical and academic background. He received his medical degree from Johns Hopkins, where he also completed a residency. Opting for a career in academic medicine, he returned to New England, where he spent nine years at Yale University as a research fellow and then as an assistant professor of internal medicine. After completing a fellowship at the University College Hospital Medical School in London, he joined the faculty at the University of Kentucky as chief of the endocrinology division. At the new and impressive medical school, Winternitz worked closely with Dean Willard, and he was influenced by Willard's belief that medical education needed to broaden its horizons beyond individual patients and their illnesses. In Tuscaloosa, Winternitz served as head of the Department of Internal Medicine and would later be appointed director of Medical Student Affairs. Winternitz proved to be a valuable addition to the teaching efforts of the College; his strength as a classical clinician and teacher who taught by example was soon recognized by students, faculty, and residents as representing the best in academic medicine. Under his direction, the Department of Internal Medicine soon became recognized for its strong and dedicated cadre of teachers.

During the same time period, Willard added several important faculty members to the Department of Community Medicine. Among these was Dr. Robert F. Gloor. Born and raised in New England, Gloor earned his medical degree from Loma Linda University in California and a Master's degree in public health from Harvard University. He joined CCHS as an associate professor of community medicine, where he directed medical students in their community medicine experience for more than twelve years until his retirement in 1988. Even after retirement he continued to serve the college until his death in 1994.

Dr. James Leeper joined the college in 1977 as the department's first non-physician member. With a degree in preventive medicine and environmental health from the University of Iowa and a concentration in biostatistics, Leeper sought to stimulate research in the college.

The addition of many well-qualified faculty members strengthened the program and an effort was made to make the college function more smoothly; in 1977 Willard and Scutchfield reorganized the college. The division of Family and Community Medicine was separated into the separate departments: the Department of Family Medicine and the Department of Community Medicine. Dr. Riley Lumpkin was asked to serve as assistant dean for continuing education and public relations. Also, a Division of Emergency Medicine was created in the Department of Surgery. It was led by Dr. Philip Bobo, the medical director of the emergency department at DCH and a dynamic teacher.

In 1977, after much had been done to upgrade the CCHS program, the LCME handed down some good news. Acknowledging the recent improvements at CCHS, the accrediting agency agreed to raise the number of students allowed at Tuscaloosa from twelve to twenty-two per year, putting the Tuscaloosa program on par with the Huntsville program. Furthermore, the LCME agreed to remove the requirement that all third-year undergraduate medical students spend the first six months of their clinical time in Birmingham. This requirement was not rescinded for students who had transferred to the program from other schools, but at least for those who had done their basic sciences training in Birmingham, there was relief.

In spite of the positive news for the medical education program in Tuscaloosa, the college's administrators could not rest. The next comprehensive review of the program was scheduled for January 1979. For more than a year prior to the LCME visit, a self-study was conducted. Hopes ran high that the accrediting agency would find fewer faults, but this was not the case.

The final report of the LCME transmitted to the UASMEP in July 1979 spelled trouble for the entire medical program in Alabama. Once again, accreditation was extended for only three years and in particular, the agency issued harsh criticism of the program in Tuscaloosa, referring to the "severe problems of this branch campus." The letter cited problems with the administrative organization, with faculty recruitment and with deteriorated academic strength. Governance issues, as before, were also cited as a problem. In the letter to Hill from LCME Secretary James R. Schofield, the school was warned that failure to comply with the Supplemental Guidelines for Branch Campuses issued by the LCME might be cause for reconsideration of the accreditation status "of the entire operation."

Many of those in the College were surprised and angered by the conclusions drawn by the members of the LCME. Willard in particular felt that the group that reviewed the program had "misjudged the situation."[55]

Knopke would later reflect on the situation with the LCME—and the frustrations associated with the negative review. "It was political as much as anything else and Willard knew it," he said, noting that Willard had served on the LCME in the past and "knew how it worked." "He thought they [Birmingham] had 'got to them,'" he said.

Willard would later claim that "results of the accreditation visit gave UAB the opportunity to obtain what it covertly wanted: control of the programs at Tuscaloosa and Huntsville."[56] Now in his last year at the University, Willard was frustrated and tired, and announced he was taking the month of July off. In fact, he would opt to retire soon thereafter.

The results of this latest review had a major repercussion on the Tuscaloosa campus. With Willard no longer at the helm and the threatened dissolution of the program, the wheels of change began to churn even more forcefully. Key administrators in UASMEP were alarmed by the report from the LCME, and it was decided before the end of the year that the board of trustees should get involved in a major overhaul of the medical education program.

5
A Change in Leadership

Nineteen seventy-nine was a difficult year for CCHS, a time when the viability of the program was threatened by a number of factors. The LCME review that had taken place in January and fiercely criticized the program had dealt a major blow to the faculty and staff of the college. Financial woes in the form of reduced allocations from the state also put pressure on the efforts of the program. Lastly, the retirement of Dr. Willard—who represented to many the heart and soul of the program—left people speculating about the future of the college. Even under the best of circumstances, the departure of a strong leader from any organization presents challenges, but Willard's departure during this tumultuous time appeared especially foreboding.

"That was a very tough time," said CCHS faculty member Dr. Robert Pieroni, reflecting on 1979, "many people left and many of us wondered if we ought to."

Willard Passes the Torch

When Dean Willard announced his intention of taking the month of July 1979 off, few people realized that he would not return as dean. At the age of seventy, Willard had reached mandatory retirement age in the University of Alabama system. He had spent the last seven years of his forty-two-year career at Alabama building the medical education program, of which he was justifiably proud. But his time as dean was winding down. The university was searching, unsuccessfully, for a successor to Willard, and in the winter of 1978–79, Vice President Thigpen asked him if he could remain in the job a bit longer.

But by July, Willard realized it was time to move on. "At that particular time I was tired and somewhat frustrated. Administrative relationships, while not bad, were not as satisfactory as they had been when I came," Willard recalled.[57] Willard was particularly frustrated by relations with his old ally, David Mathews, who now appeared "distant." In fact, Mathews was in the midst of his own crisis. The university faculty, organized around a strong and vocal Faculty Senate, was growing increasingly discontented with the administration and specifically with the president. By autumn, the group would appeal to the university's board of trustees to replace the president, and within the next year, Mathews would resign in response. The college could no longer rely on the steadfast support of David Mathews.

Nor could they continue to lean on the leader who had built the college and nurtured it for seven years. Difficult as it was, the faculty and staff of CCHS had to bid farewell to Willard as he made plans to retire to his Moundville catfish farm. He expressed no regret for having to retire, noting that the college had reached a point where it could operate better "with a different cast of characters."[58]

In speaking of Willard's accomplishments in health care and medical education in particular in Alabama, President Mathews spoke of the many contributions Willard had made, not only as an administrator, but as a mentor of people, and one who was committed to providing better health care to the citizenry.

"There is no prouder accomplishment for Bill Willard than for him to have been founder of the University's College of Community Health Sciences," said Mathews. "We at the university are grateful for his many contributions to the college, the community, the state and the nation."[59]

CCHS Assistant Dean Dr. T. Riley Lumpkin, in a letter to the editor of the *Tuscaloosa News*, wrote of Willard's contributions, noting how great an honor it was to work for a man who has "truly devoted his life to other people."[60] There was no question his presence in the college would be missed.

The Need for a New Leader

The administration in Birmingham and on the UA campus immediately set to work to identify a new leader, knowing they needed a strong leader to help guide the college through those tumultuous times. The national search for a new dean, however, went slowly, and it was obvious that they would need an interim dean while the search went on. The person who would temporarily fill Dean Willard's position needed to be someone special. The job required someone who could help mend the damage caused by the negative LCME review earlier in the year, smooth relations with the administration in Birmingham, and reassure the college faculty, staff, students, and residents in the program—who had all endured a difficult year. To do all this and continue to build on the legacy of Bill Willard was no small task. Mathews turned to Riley Lumpkin to serve as interim dean.

Lumpkin recalls that day in July, 1979, when President Mathews asked him to come to the president's office and told him that he would serve as the interim dean of the college while the search for a new dean was conducted. Although Lumpkin was somewhat reluctant to take on the job, Mathews expressed his confidence in Lumpkin's abilities. In a statement for the press, Mathews noted that Lumpkin would serve as "a calming and stabilizing factor in the transition to a new dean," noting that the new dean would have primary responsibility for working on the accreditation of the college.

Riley Lumpkin proved an excellent choice indeed for the position of interim dean. As a native of Tuskegee, Alabama, an alumnus of UA, and one of the first faculty members of the college, Lumpkin knew the system and its history very well. After college, serving in the Korean War and working toward a Master's degree in herpetology, Lumpkin also had some relevant work experience that served him well later in life: he was employed as a surgical and hospital supply salesman while in graduate school in Tuscaloosa and knew many of the doctors in the area.

When Lumpkin later decided to attend medical school, he attended UASOM in Birmingham, which granted him his medical degree in 1958. Following an internship at Mobile General Hospital, Lumpkin then entered general practice in Tuskegee. Dr. Lumpkin practiced in Tuskegee and then in Enterprise, Alabama, for a total of seventeen years before coming to the faculty full-time.

Lumpkin also had experience in administration with the college. He had served as director of the Family Practice Center when it first opened. Not long after that Dr. Willard asked him to assume responsibility for the continuing medical education program as assistant dean for Continuing Medical Education (CME). This program provides medical lectures for practicing physicians in Tuscaloosa and the surrounding towns. In Alabama each practicing physician was required to earn twelve hours of CME credit per year in order to maintain his or her license. Lumpkin's approach to CME took the shape of a daily noon lecture series for practicing physicians in the area taught by college faculty, doctors from the medical school in Birmingham, and visiting lecturers. DCH soon joined in the support of the program. National certification by the Liaison Committee on Continuing Medical Education (LCCME) soon followed.

Lumpkin was fully engaged in teaching, administration, and service to the local community when he took on the role of interim dean. It was a hard role to fill, he would soon learn. But in him the college found a sense of continuity and stability, great experience, and dedication to the principles of family practice. These traits, combined with his openness and friendliness, went a long way toward reassuring the administration in Birmingham that the problems in Tuscaloosa, whether real or merely perceived, would soon be resolved.

But even with his experience and skill, Lumpkin encountered a multitude of challenges in his newly assigned role. One of his first assignments, dispensed by President Mathews, was to relieve Dr. Scutchfield, then associate dean for Administrative Affairs, of his duties. Although many in the college assumed that Scutchfield would be Dean Willard's choice to become his successor as dean, President Mathews had other ideas. It was well known that Scutchfield would not be acceptable to Birmingham. Scutchfield's hard-charging style had offended a number of faculty members, town physicians, and medical school administrators in Birmingham. The university knew it needed someone who could build bridges, and Scutchfield clearly could not serve in that capacity. It was not long after being relieved of his title and responsibilities that he left to become director of the Graduate School of Public Health at San Diego State University in California, where he has had a distinguished career.

Another early task for Dr. Lumpkin was to pay a visit to Executive Dean Pittman, his new supervisor in Birmingham.

"Jim Pittman had nothing but criticism for me as soon as I walked in his office," recalled Lumpkin in an interview. "I think he was upset about not being involved, or even being notified or asked, about my appointment. Jim and I have been friends since I was in medical school. He was a medical resident when I was a student and his wife, Connie Pittman, taught me physical diagnosis. I responded to him, 'Jim, I'm trying to do a job and I don't know what I'm doing, and you are supposed to help me and guide me to do this thing right.' He responded and he started working with us to do some things that needed to be done."

This meeting would mark the start of improved relations between Pittman and the administration of CCHS.

The Aftermath of the 1979 LCME

One of the major issues facing Lumpkin during his tenure was, of course, the negative LCME review that took place in January 1979. When the resulting report was issued in July, the bad news quickly spread to the university's board of trustees, the state legislature, even the general public. The front page of the *Birmingham News* reported on the "severe problems" at the Tuscaloosa campus and the need to correct them quickly.[61] It was under these circumstances, with the entire program in jeopardy, that Lumpkin assumed the leadership of the college. The aftermath of the review meant Lumpkin and every aspect of the program would be scrutinized, and Lumpkin would spend the majority of his time as interim dean defending a program that he believed in, but that he was only just beginning to know how to lead.

When word of the LCME evaluation of the college—with its criticisms of the Tuscaloosa program in particular—reached the board of trustees, they immediately assumed a more active role in the medical education program. Shortly after, Lumpkin was asked to meet with the Health Affairs Committee of the board of trustees to report on the status of the college. Also present from the Tuscaloosa campus were Professor Thigpen, who was representing President Mathews, Knopke, associate dean for Academic Affairs, and Dr. David Hefelfinger, associate dean for Clinical Affairs. Dr. Lumpkin was surprised at the hostile level of interrogation by the board and he found it difficult to reassure the board that any supposed deficiencies were being corrected. Lumpkin recalled, "It was not a very pleasant meeting."

After examination of the medical education program, the board decided to undertake a complete revision of the 1972 McCall report, which outlined the structure of the new medical education program in Alabama as it was conceived in the early 1970s. In spite of complaints and concerns voiced by the Tuscaloosa administrators and faculty, DCH administrators, and the local community, board members noted an urgent need to meet LCME requirements. Led by Judge Daniel T. McCall, Jr., chair of the Health Affairs Committee and author of the original McCall report, the issue of governance was revisited in order to "resolve the accrediting problems of UASMEP, strengthen its administrative organization, clarify program objectives, and enhance the general quality of the system program."[62]

The new McCall report of 1980 was a much larger and more detailed version of the 1972 version; it was expanded from five pages to thirty pages. Several key changes were made to UA's program, starting with modification of the name of the state's medical education system. The report designated the new official name to be the University of Alabama School of Medicine (UASOM) and that the name the University of Alabama System Medical Education Program—or UASMEP—be dropped. This change thus emphasized that the medical school in Birmingham was the one medical school in the system, but with branch campuses located on the Huntsville and Tuscaloosa campuses of UA.

Another change in terminology was made in reference to the deans of each branch campus. The authors of the report changed the titles of the deans in Tuscaloosa and Huntsville to associate dean and made these individuals directly responsible to the dean of UASOM, Dr. James Pittman. Pittman would continue in his role as chief executive officer of the School of Medicine and also have increased responsibility for the branch campus programs. As such he would be responsible for selecting the associate deans at each campus and assigning their primary responsibilities. According to the report, Pittman would have to approve all full-time faculty appointments within the school and would also play a role in promotion and tenure decisions. This was a huge departure from the previous mode of operation at the Tuscaloosa and Huntsville campuses.

The report also created a new position in the system, one that gave the chancellor ultimate responsibility for the University of Alabama's medical program. Dr. Charles "Scotty" McCallum, vice president for Health Affairs at UAB, was selected to serve as assistant to the chancellor for health affairs. Pittman would now report through McCallum.

A medical doctor and dentist with a long association with the UAB program, McCallum was well suited to his new job. McCallum first joined the school to do an internship in oral surgery in 1951. He joined the dentistry faculty in 1956 while pursuing his medical degree at UAB, which he received in 1957. McCallum then served on the faculty before becoming the dean of the School of Dentistry in 1962, a post he held for fifteen years before becoming vice president for Health Affairs in 1977.

The new McCall report also made another major change to the way the branch campuses would operate by clearly outlining their main priorities, which were, according to the report "to educate and train additional primary care physicians for Alabama, particularly for the rural areas of the state." Activities outside the scope of these priorities, such as outreach residency programs or allied health initiatives, were only to be conducted with the express permission of the dean in Birmingham. Furthermore, the report stated, money that was allocated for the support of medical education and research could not be used for other purposes without prior written approval of the dean of UASOM.

The faculty and administrators in Tuscaloosa looked upon this effort with alarm. Many believed that this effort by the board had been initiated by the administrators in Birmingham who wanted to "take over" the branch campuses once and for all. Those at the Tuscaloosa campus, including Dean Emeritus Willard, who was still actively involved in college affairs, believed that "UAB fails to see the broader picture and thus misunderstands what CCHS is doing, and criticizes CCHS rather than support[ing] it."[63] Yet in spite of their protests, the new McCall report was adopted by the board in February 1980. Chancellor Joseph F. Volker urged all of the campus administrators to "move immediately to implement the report in all of its aspects."[64]

The Search for a New Dean

Meanwhile, the search for a new dean for CCHS continued, led by Pittman. Several candidates were interviewed, but those who expressed interest in the job were deemed unacceptable by either the Tuscaloosa or Birmingham administration, or both. Lumpkin continued to lead the college until a suitable candidate was found, which did not happen for a year and a half after he had accepted the appointment. During that time he continued in his unwavering support of the college and continued building community support for the program. He appeared before all types of groups, large and small, to promote the program and its goals.

By summer 1980, one person had surfaced who met the requirements of the new job. Dr. Wilmer J. Coggins was currently serving as chief of the Division of Rural Health in the Department of Community Health and Family Medicine at the University of Florida in Gainesville. With the exception of a sabbatical year at the University of Maryland, Coggins had served at the University of Florida for twenty-one years.

A native of Madison, Florida, Coggins graduated from Duke University School of Medicine in 1951 and began a residency in internal medicine at Georgetown University Hospital in Washington, D.C. His residency was interrupted by a long illness and when he recovered, he and his wife, Dr. Deborah Coggins, returned home to Florida, where he established a private practice in his hometown.

"General practice changed my life, and my view of what medicine is all about," said Coggins. "My former goals of practicing internal medicine and doing research melted away as I found general practice in a rural area to be intellectually challenging and deeply rewarding." During this time, Coggins also noted the impact one could have on a community in this capacity and was gratified by that.

However, within a few years, Coggins and his wife both felt a need to continue their residency training, which had been interrupted by his illness. Coggins joined the internal medicine residency at the University of Florida in Gainesville; this in turn led to an invitation to join the faculty, which he did in 1962. Coggins then served as an instructor of medicine and quickly rose through the ranks of the college there.

The offer to come to interview at UA was a surprise, but Coggins's interest was high. Not long before he had visited the community medicine department at the University of Kentucky while Willard was dean there, and Coggins was stimulated by the rigorous curriculum and impressive faculty.

The interview at Alabama, Coggins later recalled, was marked by stark contrasts between the Birmingham and Tuscaloosa faculties and administrators. The tone of the Tuscaloosa meeting was positive, and Coggins noted enthusiasm and a commitment to family practice. In Birmingham, however, the atmosphere was quite different: the interviewers there expressed a desire to not have "another Willard." Coggins' background in clinical medicine and private practice persuaded them that public health was not his field of interest and he was offered the job as dean of CCHS in the summer of 1980. Although Coggins and his family were reluctant to leave Gainesville after so many years, it was time to try something new, and Coggins accepted the job and agreed to be on campus in January 1981. "I was excited about the challenge," said Coggins.

Coggins was an excellent find for Alabama. His years in private practice in a rural setting combined with his experience at the University of Florida made him uniquely qualified for the task of leading the college. When he arrived on campus in January 1981, he was greeted warmly by a group of faculty and staff greatly in need of reassurance and stability. Assuming the deanship from Lumpkin, who continued to serve the college until his retirement in 1991, Coggins would serve as dean for ten years.

6
Seeking Stability

The arrival of the newest dean to CCHS was a welcome sight to many. The search to identify a new leader had taken more than a year and the need for stability was great. While Lumpkin had done an excellent job as interim dean leading the college through a stormy time, more work was needed to take the program into the future.

The program that Coggins had agreed to lead differed significantly from the program that Dr. Willard started in 1972. At the university level, a new president Dr. Joab Thomas, a graduate of Harvard University who was on the university's biology faculty, was appointed president in 1981. The same year CCHS had a permanent faculty of thirty and a cadre of more than one hundred volunteer physicians. The small number of patients that had trickled into the temporary clinic in the seventies now amounted to more than 26,000 patient visits per year. The Family Practice Center and the Educational Tower at DCH were excellent facilities that signaled the impressive growth of the program in only nine years. And although the program had recently seen tough times in the form of accreditation difficulties, Coggins was confident in the promise of the program and believed it would contribute greatly to relieving rural Alabama's shortage of primary care in general, and of family doctors specifically. The first several years of the program had resulted in a substantial ratio of students who chose residencies in family medicine. Likewise, many of the graduates of the residency program chose to enter practice in small towns and rural areas.

The most appealing aspects of CCHS, factors that influenced Coggins's decision to join the college, were the enthusiasm of the medical students and the quality of the family practice residents. On his visits to the campus, the students seemed happy to be at the college, and appreciative of their teachers. Even though the resident group was larger, at thirty-six residents, than programs he had previously experienced, they seemed individually and as a group quite mature and serious about their work. The residency director, Dr. Samuel Gaskins, emphasized that applicants to the program would have responsibilities to teach the medical students on their service in the hospital. If an applicant preferred not to work with medical students, he or she was not welcome at CCHS.

Gaskins took pride in the fact that the attrition rate in the residency program was quite low. Coggins agreed that this was commendable while noting that some residency programs were too slow to advise the occasional underperformer to go elsewhere.

The stability of the Department of Family Medicine with Dr. Russell Anderson as chair and Gaskins directing the residency was very helpful in allowing Coggins to focus on other departments where faculty changes were more frequent.

Establishing Priorities

Dean Coggins approached his new position with a desire to get the program back on track. As he viewed the task, he noticed some areas that needed immediate attention. The first was the emphasis on outreach at a time when the medical student program was in trouble with the LCME. Although as a former family practitioner Coggins agreed with the ideals of family medicine as espoused by Willard, his first concern—and priority—was ensuring the quality of the third and fourth years of medical school on the Tuscaloosa campus.

"I firmly believed in the goals that Dean Willard and the others had established for the college, and the challenge for me was to find the best way to implement those goals," said Coggins. "I was certain that the principles on which the college were founded were sound, but the ultimate configuration of the college was still to be determined."

With encouragement from Dean Pittman and the administrators in Birmingham, the administration set out to realign the priorities of the program. Reestablishing a quality medical education program would be a main focus, and, Coggins decided, outreach activities would take a back seat for the immediate future. Charles W. Scott ("Bill"), then deputy dean of UASOM, proved to be instrumental in helping Coggins and Ficken, then director of Medical Student Affairs, establish the number of medical students he assigned to Tuscaloosa each year.

The many service programs and outreach activities Willard had set in motion outside the university were important and all could potentially contribute to improving the health care of the citizens of Alabama. Projects such as the establishment of the Maude Whatley clinic and the family practice residency in Selma affected health care in the region, and Coggins recognized their value. But a dearth of funding and a need to get the accreditation of the college settled meant that CCHS would have to pursue fewer of these projects for the foreseeable future. Furthermore, even without funding concerns, Coggins had reservations about the extent to which a medical education program could productively establish and staff clinics, or office practices, in underserved areas of the state for use as sites for medical education. Instead of establishing stand-alone clinics, he opted to use the established rural practices with doctors interested in teaching students or supervising residents in more limited numbers. "We were fortunate to have a small number in nearby communities who did that well," said Coggins (Appendices C and D).

While some on the faculty expressed regret about the change in direction that the college was taking, fearing that the original mission of the college would be lost, most realized the importance of bolstering the commitments to the medical students and residents.

The second priority for the college administrators concerned the Family Practice Center, which would be renamed the Capstone Medical Center in 1982.[65] This relatively new one-story contemporary building had an outer covering of large panels of a stone-aggregate material. This new building material was touted as a long-wearing, low-maintenance exterior surface that would not require painting. Unfortunately, by 1981, it would require much more: the sides of the building were beginning to peel off, leaving a sickly blue surface. Large, expensive repairs were required. This was especially worrisome as the school tried to improve its reputation with many key groups, including the LCME.

"It seems to me that those various publics that were important to the college might think symbolically and equate the deteriorating exterior of the major patient care and teaching building with the status of the college itself," said Coggins.

Unfortunately, repair of the building was being delayed by legal issues. The university had been unable to identify those contractors from whom to demand redress. But Coggins felt that this could not wait until the issue was resolved in court, and he appealed to the board of trustees and the vice president for Financial Affairs, Robert A. Wright. With their support, the repairs were made as the legal transactions continued.

Securing the Finances of the College

One of the biggest challenges confronting the new dean related to the finances of the college. In September 1982 the seven-year grant from the Veterans Administration would expire, which meant a loss of almost one million dollars each year to the budget of the college. One of the obvious ways to replace that money was by capturing some percentage of the patient fee income at the Capstone Medical Center (CMC) for use by CCHS. Virtually all medical schools, both public and private, had developed nonprofit entities to accomplish similar goals. Traditionally, medical school faculty had been indifferent to the income that could be generated by patients under their supervision. In urban centers with large charity hospitals, medical schools provided much of the medical care in order to have access to indigent patients for teaching purposes. However, as new medical schools evolved, and private and community hospitals joined the educational efforts, many more patients with health insurance (or Medicare and Medicaid) were served by faculty physicians. The result was a major increase in revenue for academic medical centers and as a result, faculty practice plans came into being.[66] These nonprofit organizations served as valuable administrative vehicles for faculty practices, providing multiple benefits at a time when educational costs strained medical school budgets. For example, the faculty practice plans could be used to supplement the fixed, noncompetitive salaries of faculty and provide additional fringe benefits. Such compensation would be the key to successful recruitment efforts nationwide, since faculty salaries often lagged behind physician incomes in the private sector.

Such concerns were also reflected in CCHS and by June 1981, the college had organized its own faculty practice plan called the Capstone Health Services Foundation. Designated as a nonprofit 501(c)3 organization with its own board of directors and a small management staff, the foundation was built on a model similar to the one in Birmingham, allowing for the collection of patient fee income generated by clinical faculty. The money collected, which is free of control by the university, is used to supplement clinical faculty salaries and fringe benefits, as well as patient care services when state funds are insufficient. Furthermore, patient fee income can be used to purchase new equipment and supplies for the medical center. This has often proved to be critical during those years when state funds have been limited and allocations to higher education have been reduced.

Within a year the foundation had started earning its keep. By fiscal year 1982–83 the foundation's contribution to the educational programs in Tuscaloosa was $1.1 million whereas state support of the program in that same fiscal year equaled only $3.36 million. Tremendous growth would be seen for years to come: by 1987 the clinic had seen more than 64,000 patients and the income doubled; by 2001 more than 75,000 patient encounters were recorded and patient revenue had more than doubled again. Today the foundation contributes 38 percent of the college's annual budget.

"The establishment of the foundation was extremely important to the college. Dr. Coggins's initiative in setting that up was a really good thing for us," said Dr. Roland Ficken in an interview.

Another source of potential funding at this time was DCH, with whom the college had developed a partnership to provide medical education in Tuscaloosa. Although reluctant at first to partake in the endeavor, the medical staff at the hospital was playing a prominent role by the time the college entered its second decade. However, in spite of the verbal support of the hospital and medical staff, financial support had been very limited. This contrasted with most other community teaching hospitals in the nation, which made a major contribution to medical schools in return for the services of the schools' residents and clinical faculty. The federal government typically pays hospitals for partaking in educational activities; a portion of this funding is typically passed on to the medical schools. Although it was not clear how much DCH was receiving from the federal government, the CCHS administration was sure it was at least enough to help pay resident salaries. CCHS administrators reasoned that the college provided a great deal to the hospital, helping it to meet the enormous demands for hospital coverage. CCHS faculty and residents provide patient care for many patients, including almost all of the indigent patients and assisting many of the medical staff members in their care of patients of the specialty services in the hospital. Determined to have the hospital take more responsibility for the education programs that were conducted under its roof, Coggins negotiated with the administrator at the hospital, Mr. James Ford, for $125,000 during his first year, and the hospital agreed to supply those funds. This income helped defray the cost of salaries for the first-year residents and helped make up the money in the soon-to-be terminated VA grant. By the end of Coggins's tenure in 1991, this money would slowly increase to almost $500,000 per year. While this sum represented less than many hospitals contributed toward the services of their resident physicians, the support helped the financially strained college meet its goals.

The progress made in medical education in the 1980s and in Tuscaloosa in particular is even more impressive when one considers the economic climate of the time. By 1986, Coggins's fifth year as dean, he and his staff had endured several years of reduced and prorated budgets. During the 1986–87 fiscal year, for example, the budget of the college was reduced by 11 percent and then further reduced another 5 percent later in the year. Fortunately, an increase in patient care revenue, combined with a steady increase in grants from federal and state agencies as well as private foundations, helped to offset the budget shortfalls.

Research Efforts in CCHS

Income from research grants was significant over the years and increased in spite of the small size of the faculty. In 1985, for example, six projects were funded for a total of $760,000, in addition to funding from the Ford Foundation for a study of rural Alabama pregnancies and infant health and from the Josiah Macy, Jr. Foundation for a program called BioPrep. At the time, the Macy grant was the largest private foundation grant ever received by UA in its history.

Established in 1982, the Biomedical Sciences Preparation Program, or BioPrep, evolved into an important program for the college. This high school academic honors program was the brainchild of Harry Knopke, then associate dean for Academic Affairs, and Dr. Robert Northrup, chair of the CCHS Department of Community Medicine, who established this program in an attempt to increase the number of students from rural and often disadvantaged communities who would choose careers in the health care field.

The program, which was a joint effort between the college and area high schools, included a three-pronged approach. First, it aimed to increase the students' academic competency in some key subject areas, including mathematics and science. Secondly, the program expanded the students' knowledge of the nation's health care system and the many career opportunities available. Thirdly, the program planners sought to expand the students' appreciation for the rural environments in which they were raised. The hope was that some day they would return to these areas as adults.

The program also included special activities that supplemented the curriculum, including workshops on the university campus, field trips, and field placements. All such activities were intended to "extend the students' awareness of the range of applications of their academic knowledge, to introduce them to topics and experiences not usually accessible to a rural high school student."[67]

The program was very popular with students and the participating school systems. The pilot program that was launched early in the decade with five schools had expanded to include thirty-four schools and was still growing. In 1986, with interest in the program very high in Alabama, the Macy grant was extended for four more years. The Henry J. Kaiser Foundation of California also granted funds for the continuation and expansion of the program, and state funds were later added to the mix.

The expanded program allowed for more teacher development. Teachers from the participating schools attended workshops at UA to reinforce their teaching skills for the more demanding curriculum. Enthusiasm among the faculty of the area schools was very high and attrition, consequently, was very low. Many teachers were stimulated to write grant proposals to obtain funds to purchase equipment and supplies for their schools.

The progress of the students who participated in BioPrep was followed and their success soon became clear. The averages of the American College Testing Program scores by the BioPrep students exceeded the norms of the state and the nation. By the late 1980s the program planners were able to boast that all of its students were attending college, and 74 percent of these were receiving academic scholarships. It was not long before this success brought national attention to the BioPrep program. Many school systems appealed to be admitted to the program. "The program," explained Knopke, "had established a connection with the local schools and had a good reputation. It also brought lots of visibility for UA."

As a result, efforts were made to make it available nationally. Working with faculty from UA's College of Communication and Information Sciences and personnel from the State Board of Education, BioPrep staff members established a distance learning program relating to the health sciences using satellite technology. Ultimately, a grant from the U.S. Department of Education helped this collegial effort form a new entity, the Center for Communication and Educational Technology (CCET). Led by Dr. Larry Rainey, who played a key role in BioPrep throughout its eight years, the CCET has become a permanent center, providing distance learning at the high school level to students in rural high schools across the nation.

Much of the external funding coming into the college during the 1980s could be credited to a new effort designed to provide support to ongoing research: the CCHS Research Consulting Laboratory. As CCHS was being formed as a place for educating medical students and family practice residents, it was recognized that a truly academic enterprise would also include a research component. Therefore, it was decided that researchers and research support staff needed to be recruited. On the faculty side, research expertise was concentrated in the departments of Community Medicine and Behavioral Science with Ph.D. and M.D./M.P.H. trained personnel. Faculty members of the clinical departments had research training varying from none to a fair amount. Support for these individuals was needed in order to be successful in obtaining grants and assisting clinical faculty, medical students, and residents in their research. In the college, a research committee had been formed in the 1970s with responsibility for stimulating research and developing research plans. This committee was also provided with funds to award to faculty for small projects.

In 1984, however, as the college moved forward in its efforts to strengthen its research component, Dr. James Leeper realized more was needed. He proposed to Coggins the formation of a consulting laboratory that would formalize and give visibility to the research enterprise within CCHS. The laboratory was established on the fourth floor of the Russell Student Health Center.

Initially, Dr. Leeper served as director of the lab with part-time staff, including a graduate student assistant and a keypunch operator, Marie Smith, who taught herself and became the first personal computer expert in CCHS. In the mid-1980s, Dr. Robert Pieroni of the internal medicine/family medicine faculty donated an Apple personal computer, which was a novelty at the time.

In 1989 Dr. M. Christine Nagy, who had been working as research director on a major Ford Foundation grant in CCHS for several years, was hired as the first full-time director of the Research Consulting Lab. Her full-time status allowed her the time for much more extensive outreach to CCHS faculty and others. Shortly after her tenure began, the Research Consulting Laboratory was renamed the Health Research Consulting Service (HRCS), to make it more descriptive of its activities.

Improvements on the Accreditation Front

The redefinition of and improvements in the Tuscaloosa program were reflected in the next LCME reviews. In a required August 1982 progress report from the School of Medicine to the LCME, the improvements could already be seen. The report claimed to be in full compliance with the McCall report of 1980 and addressed the improved communication and cooperation between the parent campus and the branch campus. The report also noted the increase in research activities and grants received and the filling of some key positions, including the chief of family medicine at CCHS. The report further noted that the focus of the Tuscaloosa program was now firmly fixed on providing high quality educational experiences for students and residents and "less on extramural community service programs."[68]

Another key indication of the significant enhancements that had been made in the educational arena in Tuscaloosa could be seen in the objective test scores of the third-year medical students at Tuscaloosa. A study of the performances across each of the three clinical clerkship sites (Birmingham, Huntsville, and Tuscaloosa) in the required clerkships in internal medicine, obstetrics/gynecology, pediatrics, psychiatry, and surgery indicated that Tuscaloosa students did at least as well as their counterparts at the other sites. In fact, Tuscaloosa students in three of the five subject areas scored significantly higher than at either of the other campuses. CCHS administrators, faculty, and staff had reason to be proud.

The next major test of the CCHS program and the progress it was making was during the October 1984 comprehensive review by the LCME of the UASOM program. For the first time since he came to UA, Dean Coggins could be fully involved in the review. After four days of scrutiny by the review team, the members of the team reported that they were favorably impressed with the progress made at all three campuses. Although they did recommend some areas for improvements, they also noted several specific positive developments, including the increased levels of financial support that had been developed at UASOM, the well-managed clinical services program, and the high quality of the faculty and staff. The team also noted, "with approbation," the large number of graduates who had entered primary care positions, particularly within the state. The faculty and staff in Tuscaloosa were gratified by this observation.

In June 1985 the medical school received its official accreditation report. This time the LCME conferred full accreditation on the program for a six-year period and permitted the School of Medicine to admit 165 students, rather than the previous limitation of 150. For the first time since the college was opened, the administrators felt some relief from the constant visits, self-studies, and reviews that they had undergone by the LCME. Such activities consumed a great deal of time and effort. When in 1985, the college administrators learned the program would not undergo another major review until the 1990–91 academic year, there was a general sense of relief. When the next LCME review took place in 1990, the last one during Coggins's tenure, the outcome was even more impressive. This time accreditation was extended for seven years. Particularly satisfying to the CCHS faculty and administration were the team's laudatory remarks about the branch campuses in Tuscaloosa and Huntsville during their exit interview. A major hurdle had been cleared.

Physical Growth and Improvements

On top of the improvements being made to the college in the areas of education and administration, key enhancements were also made to the physical holdings of the college. From the beginning of his tenure, Coggins sought to enhance the excellent facilities built for CCHS. "We had some superb facilities, but as a group we were too spread out," said Coggins. "My immediate goal was to get our faculty as close to one location as possible."

To that end, Coggins immediately made a plea to top UA officials that a new facility be built to house all the faculty, staff and administrators. In 1981 a request for more than $3 million in capital funds was made to UA president Thomas for the construction of faculty and administrative offices adjacent to the Family Practice Center.

While waiting for the administration's decision, Coggins focused on making improvements to the clinic. Soon after the exterior was repaired additional steps were taken toward expanding it. The center had long been the centerpiece of the clinical teaching program, but it was too small for the growing college's needs and had been almost since its inception. The steady increase in patient visits that had occurred since the college was founded led to the use of five double-wide trailers for clinical activities. Set directly behind the clinic in 1974 as the facility was under construction, these temporary facilities were wholly inadequate: they were too hot in the summer months and too cool in the winter. During thunderstorms or when tornado warnings were issued, everyone in the trailers had to move into the main building for safety reasons. Furthermore, their distance from the clinic's laboratory and x-ray facilities made the trailers inconvenient for patients and the staff. By the time Coggins was leading CCHS, gathering all the patient care activities into one location had became a priority, and renovation and expansion seemed the best way to accomplish this goal. The CCHS administrators knew that large and expensive changes would lead to greater comfort and convenience for the patients, an enhanced appearance for the clinic, and would also help the college's standing with the accrediting agencies.

The work on the Family Practice Center, renamed the Capstone Medical Center the same year that this construction was begun, was done in two phases and added more than seven thousand square feet of clinical space to the facility. With construction beginning in 1982, the first enhancement was the renovation of space formerly occupied by the State Forensic Science Laboratory. The forensics staff was using the area for storage, and Coggins appealed to have the group relocated. After several months Dr. Roger Sayers, then vice president for Academic Affairs and later president, found space elsewhere for the displaced state forensics personnel. Renovation of this office was paid for in part by a grant from the federal Department of Health and Human Services, and by November of 1983, the Business Office was moved here, thus making room in the CMC for the new Blue Suite, one of three devoted to family practice.

In 1984 work started on the addition of a new "supersuite," the Red Suite, which would house two of the four medical teams for family practice. It was opened in summer 1985 and added four thousand square feet of space, including a new waiting room, fifteen new examining rooms and a minor surgery/procedures room to the CMC. The addition of the new suite reduced the number of family medicine suites from three smaller suites to two larger, more efficient units.

In November of the same year, a new Ob/Gyn suite was ready for use. This fifteen-hundred-foot area, formerly used by the family medicine department, included six examining rooms, facilities for gynecological surgical procedures, and a reception area that allowed for more privacy for patients. All combined, the many changes at the CMC represented the positive growth of the program.

But the improvements that were taking place on the CMC's physical structure were not the only ones. In 1985 the clinic, under the leadership of administrator George Tulli, became the nation's first university-sponsored, non-hospital-based outpatient clinic to be accredited by the Joint Commission on Accreditation of Hospitals and Ambulatory Health Services. Accreditation by the agency was considered by many to be a benchmark of quality and involved a review of the CMC standards of administration, quality of care, medical records, and a host of other requirements. Among these was the implementation of a quality assurance program that would establish specific goals for improvement, to be reviewed periodically by a committee of doctors, residents, nurses, and support staff that came in contact with patients. Additional, increasingly ambitious goals were added periodically. This was a major departure from the CMC's former approach to quality, which consisted of monthly patient chart reviews by doctors, residents, and medical records personnel.

One of the last major changes to the CCHS facilities was made in 1990 at the Medical Education Tower at DCH. The auditorium on the first floor, the largest educational space in the college, was, under hospital administrator Ford's leadership, remodeled and upgraded to better suit the needs of both college and hospital personnel. The renovation was generously supported by individual contributions by friends of the College and DCH, which also used the room for a variety of educational programs. The remodeled auditorium was renamed the William R. Willard Auditorium, in honor of the founding dean, and a large dedication ceremony was held with Willard in attendance. Today the facility continues to be used almost daily.

Additional Threats to the Program

During the 1980s CCHS underwent great changes as the program was first steadied, and then slowly evolved. But as relations with Birmingham improved and accreditation issues subsided, new threats to the future of the program arose; by 1984, the program was again threatened, but this time CCHS was not singled out. Some national studies, including a major report issued by the Graduate Medical Education National Advisory Committee in 1980, suggested that too many physicians were being produced. Many warned that a soon-to-occur excess number of doctors would add to the rising cost of medical care.

To some, the cost of medical education in Alabama seemed excessive and a governor's task force on economic recovery was convened by then Governor Fob James. Chaired by UAB President Hill, the committee recommended reducing the number of graduating physicians to a more "realistic level."[69] To that end, the committee stated that maintenance of the three-campus medical education program was neither practical nor cost effective. Their recommendations stood in sharp contrast to the data that suggested that Alabama was still suffering from a chronic lack of primary care physicians, particularly in rural areas. A 1984 study by Willard and his colleagues Dr. Elizabeth Ruben and Dr. Harry Knopke reported that Alabama was still far short of its goal to provide one primary care physician for every one thousand persons. This compelling data revealed that the maldistribution of doctors in the state's rural areas still posed a threat to accessible health care.[70]

These same findings would be echoed several years later in a study by Dean Coggins and Colleen Beall, a research associate in the CCHS geriatrics program. Their 1988 study employed health manpower resource data furnished by the State Health Planning Agency for Alabama and found that overall, Alabama continued to suffer from a serious medical manpower shortage. Although the ratio of physician to population had improved over the past decade, the authors said, "it is apparent that Alabama as a whole continues to be underserved."

"Each physician in the state must serve on average, thirty-seven percent more patients than the figure determined as optimal, assuming utilization rates equal to the national average. Even this picture, however, is misleading because those physicians are not distributed evenly across that state."[71] Furthermore, the authors expressed a fear that the trend would worsen as older general practitioners retired from their rural practices and younger physicians continued to seek employment in the state's urban areas.

The university's board of trustees, however, elected to undertake a study to examine the medical school and its two branch campuses, based on the findings of the governor's task force. The CCHS contribution to the report consisted of a forty-page summary of its educational programs and expenditures of state and grant funds. The time and effort required to prepare such a document were burdensome, coming as they did, when the accreditation reports were due so frequently. Yet the resulting documentation gave those in Tuscaloosa a feeling of satisfaction as they reflected on the many accomplishments that had occurred over such a short time.

As the report neared completion, the three campuses were given one week to make comments on the final document. Coggins noted how much effort was required to make cool, rational comments when the final outcome may have resulted in a death sentence for the program. In March 1984 the board announced a decision to adopt the report that recommended a 25 percent cut in the number of students admitted to Alabama's medical school annually. They looked to Governor Wallace, who was in office again from 1983–87, to take the next step. Wallace, however, announced his disagreement with the findings of the report, noting that not every person in the state had ready access to quality medical care. He told reporters, "I want to see a time in Alabama when they (doctors) will advertise in the Clayton Record (the governor's hometown newspaper), 'We make house calls on Sunday.'"[72] The board thus decided not to change the structure of the state's medical programs nor to reduce its enrollment. Although this would not be the last threat to the branch campuses in Tuscaloosa and Huntsville, no more was heard about the issue at that time.

It was not until 1990 that the college would have to endure another attempt to dismantle the program; this time the threat came from Birmingham. That year Dean Pittman announced his consideration of a plan to rotate all students to Tuscaloosa or Huntsville, so that none would be placed at either campus for the full two years. Although Bill Scott, as deputy dean of UASOM, assured the faculty in Tuscaloosa that such a plan was unworkable, the faculty felt threatened. Coggins in particular was disappointed by this latest move to undermine the medical student program. He had worked for almost ten years to ensure the quality and stability of the medical student program and reviews of the program by the students were quite positive, emphasizing the direct teaching by the faculty in all of the rotations. Although this consideration by Pittman did not materialize, it demonstrated just how uncertain the position of the college could be.

The HMO Experiment

One of the big changes to health care that took place during the 1980s was the growing popularity of health maintenance organizations (HMOs). These organizations were conceived of in the United States during the Nixon administration in an attempt to improve the capacity and efficiency of the nation's burgeoning health system. Long touted as a major advance in the organization and delivery of health care, HMOs provide medical care on a prepaid basis and emphasize outpatient care and preventive health services, such as immunizations and regular screenings for serious illnesses. Employing primary care physicians as the doctor of record for every patient is said to improve efficiency and lead to increased cost savings. The major constraint in the system is that the HMO will pay for the services of a specialist only if the primary care physician, the gatekeeper, approves. HMOs also introduced a concept that was considered radical by U.S. standards, that of paying a fixed annual fee for each patient assigned to the physician, regardless of how often the doctor sees the patient. In this situation, the physician shares the risks of excessive use by the patients with the HMO.

The first HMO to arrive in Tuscaloosa was HealthAmerica, a large provider based in Harrisburg, Pennsylvania. After extensive study and deliberation, the foundation contracted with HealthAmerica in 1985. The clinical faculty and staff entered into this new scheme with interest; very few had experience with HMOs, which were rapidly gaining in popularity around the country. Coggins believed that this venture would give the faculty and residents valuable experience with the HMO model, even though it put an additional burden on the family medicine department.

When HealthAmerica began business in Tuscaloosa, more than two hundred patients chose to receive their primary care at the CMC; they were virtually all new patients. The physicians disliked having to play the role of gatekeeper when the occasional patient demanded to see a specialist without the approval of their primary physician. Monthly lump sums from the HMO were made to the CMC, and these were often slow in coming.

After two years, HealthAmerica opted to discontinue its contract in Tuscaloosa, citing a low enrollment. In the parlance of the health economists, they had "withdrawn from the local market." Although the clinic had not reaped huge financial benefits from the arrangement, the administrators soon realized a hidden cost of this experiment: the loss of continuity of care for so many individuals.

"This event was very disruptive for both the patient and doctor," recalled Coggins. "Familiarity and trust is mutually beneficial in the doctor-patient relationship and the disruption for 'market' considerations cannot be measured in dollars. We had learned a valuable lesson."

Addition of Nontenured Faculty Positions

By the late 1980s there was pressure for the CCHS faculty to devote more time to the teaching programs, to direct patient care, and to perform and publish research as the path to promotion and tenure. As a result it became clear that not all faculty could conduct true research. Although the college could reasonably expect them to support the research of others or to write reports for publication, not all were able to conceptualize, find funding, pursue the research, analyze the data, and publish the results. Because the faculty was subject to promotion and tenure guidelines of the university, Coggins sought to develop a nontenure or so-called clinical track for outstanding teachers who were also committed to patient care. At the main campus in Birmingham, no formalized system existed outside of the traditional promotion and tenure track, although it was clear that valued teachers and productive patient care faculty were not forced to leave. As such, without a model from UASOM, college administrators studied the guidelines of five other medical schools, all in the top ten in the country, in order to formulate the new rules. The main consideration was that the nontenure track could not be used as an escape hatch, allowing faculty members who reached the tenure deadline to suddenly change tracks. Establishing the system was not difficult, Coggins recalled, since the university administration appreciated the problem. This arrangement has allowed many good teachers who are committed to patient care to continue their careers while the volume of research continues to increase.

The Impact of AIDS at UA

One of the primary functions of any medical program is to serve a community, and CCHS was able to play a larger role in this respect when AIDS first made its appearance on the UA campus in 1987. At the time there was widespread fear and public misunderstanding about the disease, which had only first been described in the medical literature in 1981. Questions about how it was acquired, how it was transmitted, and how it might be treated were raised. When the disease first began to appear in young people, its association with sexual activity and illegal drug use suggested that some individuals in college populations might be at increased risk. Colleges and universities across the country found the threat of AIDS among their students, staff, and faculty particularly threatening and were concerned about their legal status in respect to "victims' rights" (admission and retention of students, hiring and retention of staff) versus legitimate concerns about new infection by direct contact or body fluids.

President Thomas recognized that UA must confront the threat since it was likely the university would have a student with AIDS on campus at some time and there were possible issues with the faculty and staff. In November the president appointed a committee cochaired by Coggins to study the implications that students with AIDS would have on all aspects of the university and to recommend a policy for the university. In the meantime, Dr. Winternitz, Dr. Coggins, and Dr. Mary Sawyer, a CCHS faculty member with experience in infectious diseases—in concert with the personnel office and the university's legal group—gave a series of lectures to the university staff and faculty to educate them about the risks of the virus.

Not long after the committee was formed, an article in the *Crimson White*, UA's student newspaper, disclosed that a university staff member was infected with HIV. This focused the attention of the committee, which—after studying similar documents from other institutions, especially that at the University of Virginia—developed an AIDS policy for the university. Thomas accepted the policy, which then went before the board of trustees for approval. The policy was adopted in spring 1988.

Education of the medical student and resident populations about HIV/AIDS also became a high priority. Concerns about the health of students, residents, and the patients they would come in contact with were great. Many conferences and educational seminars were given to help educate these future medical professionals about this disease.

Educational efforts were also undertaken by the CCHS Health Sciences Library. The director of the library, Lisa Rains Russell, and her staff recognized the need for information, not just for the health professional, but for the general public. Consequently, the library staff developed an AIDS information center that consisted of scientific papers, informational brochures, and audiovisual material that was available to university personnel and the general public.[73] In this way the college was able to contribute to the community as it dealt with the many issues surrounding the growing AIDS epidemic. Fortunately, accurate diagnostic tests and the discovery of partially effective treatments came along rapidly, and AIDS did not become a serious problem for the university.

The End of an Era

In late 1990 Dean Coggins announced his retirement. A series of health problems and a realization that he had been dean for ten years led to the decision.

"I felt that a number of concerns from 1981 had been resolved. The medical student program was secure and highly regarded by a sufficient number of students in Birmingham and the family residency program was very successful," he said.

Coggins knew that a new, energetic and imaginative leader was needed to address the new problems associated with the new initiatives in the college. His only concern as he departed was the clear need for more space for patient care, teaching, and faculty accommodations, but Coggins was certain this would be resolved in time.

When Coggins departed in January 1991, Pittman asked Dr. Roland Ficken to serve as interim dean while a search was conducted. It was to mark another chapter in the history of CCHS.

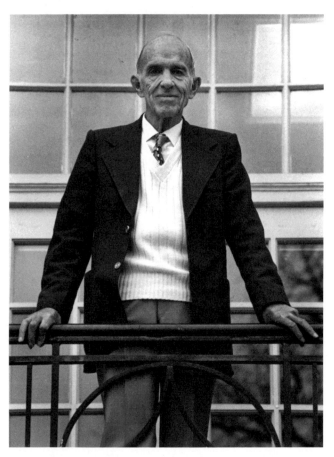

Dean William R. Willard
Dr. William R. Willard was the founding dean of the college and
a leading figure in establishing the field of family medicine.

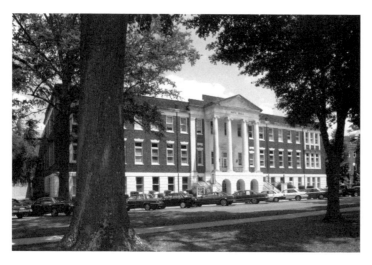

Nott Hall

Nott Hall was named for Dr. Josiah Nott, the well-respected surgeon and medical leader in Mobile who founded the first medical school there. It housed a two-year medical program in Tuscaloosa from 1920 to 1945 before it was moved to Birmingham to become the UA School of Medicine. Nott Hall has housed administrative and faculty offices for the college since 1974.

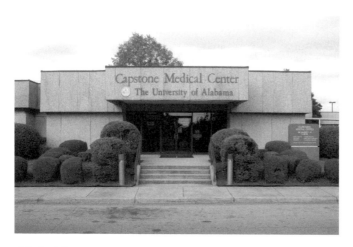

Capstone Medical Center

The Capstone Medical Center, built across the street from DCH Regional Medical Center in 1975, is the main clinical facility for the college.

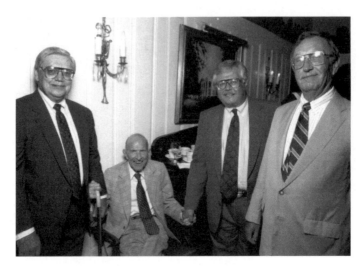

Former Deans of the College
[from left to right] Dr. Riley T. Lumpkin, Interim Dean 1979–80; Dr. William R. Willard, Dean 1973–79; Dr. Roland P. Ficken, Dean 1990–95; Dr. Wilmer J. Coggins, Dean 1980–90.

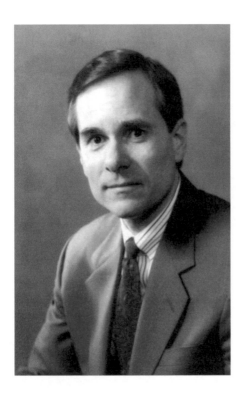

Dr. William C. Curry
Fourth and current dean of the college, appointed in 1998 after a distinguished career in private practice in Carrollton, Alabama. While in private practice, Dr. Curry served more than twenty years as an adjunct member of the college's internal medicine faculty.

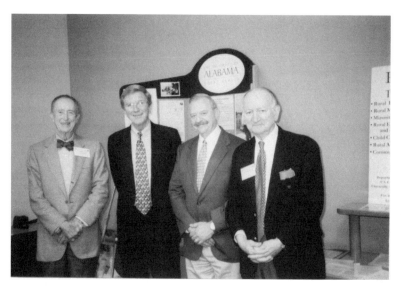

Founding Fathers
[From left to right] Dr. John Burnum, Dr. David Mathews, Dr. William
Owings, and Dr. Richard Rutland, shown at the 2002 Rural Health Confer-
ence, were instrumental in the founding of the college.

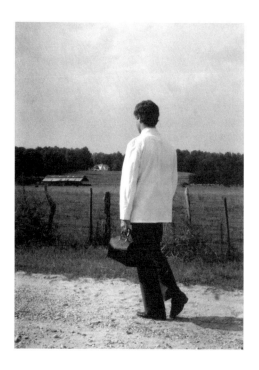

Medical Student Sage Smith
This picture of Sage Smith, a
former medical student who
now practices in Monroeville,
Alabama, is used as a symbol of
the college's rural health programs. The picture was taken at
a farm in northern Tuscaloosa
County in the early 1980s.

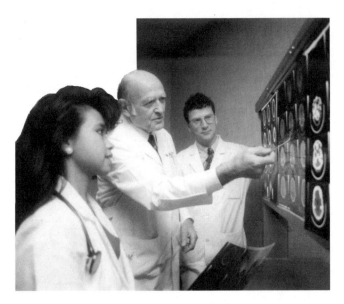

Dr. William W. Winternitz and Medical Students
Medical students with Dr. William Winternitz, longtime chairman of the department of Internal Medicine.

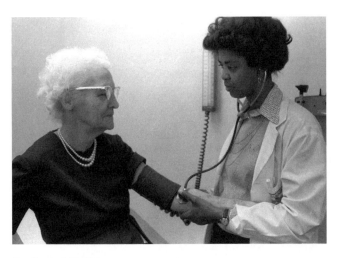

Dr. Sandral Hullett
Dr. Sandral Hullett, shown examining a patient, completed the Family Practice Residency in 1979. Hullett served as the medical director of West Alabama Health Services for many years and garnered a national reputation for her expertise in rural health. She served on the Board of Trustees of the University of Alabama System from November 1982 to September 2001.

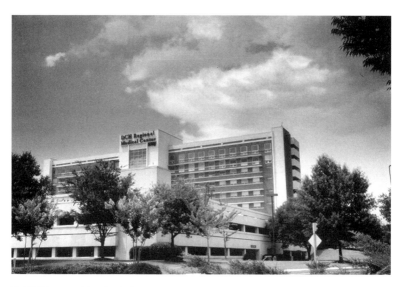

DCH Regional Medical Center
Opened in 1952 as the 240-bed Druid City Hospital, additions between 1958 and 1976 brought DCH to 496 beds. The opening of a five-story wing in 1976 made DCH the state's third largest hospital. DCH serves as partner for the Family Practice Residency and the inpatient teaching facility for the college.
(*photograph by Tim Martin*)

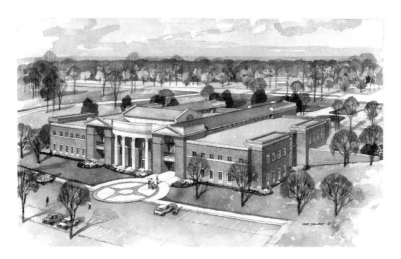

CCHS's New Building
Groundbreaking was held in November 2002 for the College's new home, a 77,000-square foot facility that will combine all of the college's academic activities in one location for the first time in thirty years. It is scheduled for occupancy in May 2004.

University of Alabama School of Medicine - Tuscaloosa
College of Community Health Sciences
Practice Sites of Family Practice Residents / Medical Student Graduates

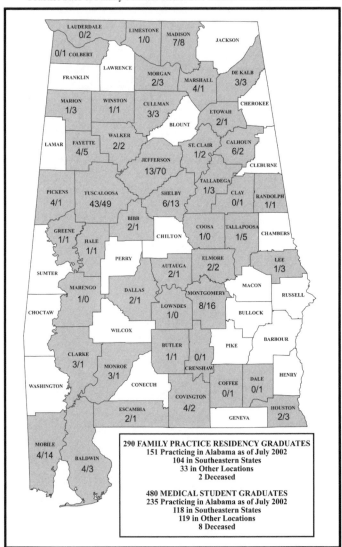

LAUDERDALE 0/2
LIMESTONE 1/0
MADISON 7/8
JACKSON
0/1 COLBERT
LAWRENCE
FRANKLIN
MORGAN 2/3
MARSHALL 4/1
DE KALB 3/3
MARION 1/3
WINSTON 1/1
CULLMAN 3/3
ETOWAH 2/1
CHEROKEE
BLOUNT
WALKER 2/2
LAMAR
FAYETTE 4/5
ST. CLAIR 1/2
CALHOUN 6/2
JEFFERSON 13/70
CLEBURNE
TALLADEGA 1/3
PICKENS 4/1
TUSCALOOSA 43/49
SHELBY 6/13
CLAY 0/1
RANDOLPH 1/1
BIBB 2/1
GREENE 1/1
HALE 1/1
CHILTON
COOSA 1/0
TALLAPOOSA 1/5
CHAMBERS
PERRY
AUTAUGA 2/1
ELMORE 2/2
LEE 1/3
SUMTER
MARENGO 1/0
DALLAS 2/1
MONTGOMERY 8/16
MACON
RUSSELL
CHOCTAW
LOWNDES 1/0
BULLOCK
WILCOX
CLARKE 3/1
MONROE 3/1
BUTLER 1/1
PIKE 0/1
CRENSHAW
BARBOUR
WASHINGTON
CONECUH
COFFEE 0/1
DALE 0/1
HENRY
COVINGTON 4/2
ESCAMBIA 2/1
GENEVA
HOUSTON 2/3
MOBILE 4/14
BALDWIN 4/3

290 FAMILY PRACTICE RESIDENCY GRADUATES
151 Practicing in Alabama as of July 2002
104 in Southeastern States
33 in Other Locations
2 Deceased

480 MEDICAL STUDENT GRADUATES
235 Practicing in Alabama as of July 2002
118 in Southeastern States
119 in Other Locations
8 Deceased

Alumni Map of Alabama
As of July 2002, there were 209 graduates of the Family Practice Residency and
480 medical student graduates. This map depicts the practice location of the 151
residency graduates and the 235 medical student graduates in Alabama.

7
The Program Emerges

When Roland Ficken became the interim dean of CCHS, the college was approaching its twentieth year. During that time the program had seen a great deal of turmoil: budgetary cuts, conflicts with UASOM, and threats to the program all created challenges for the faculty and administration. But in spite of the times of uncertainty, one thing was irrefutable: the college was fulfilling its mission of training primary care doctors and placing them in the state's rural areas and small towns. By 1991 more than 251 medical students had completed the two-year clinical program and 23 percent of these had chosen careers in family practice (compared to a national average of just 12 percent). Likewise, 165 residents had completed the family practice residency program in Tuscaloosa (Appendix A) and of these, more than half were practicing in Alabama, many in small towns or rural areas. The college could proudly claim to have one of the most productive family practice residencies in the country, being in the top 10 percent in the number of residents graduated. By fall 1991 a permanent leader was needed who could anticipate the ever-changing challenges in medical education and medical care and who could confront the ever-present shortage of funds for public education in Alabama.

Identifying a New Dean

Ficken served as interim dean for seven months before he was approached about taking the position on a more permanent basis. The search committee formed to find a new dean for CCHS had failed to find a promising candidate for the post after a national search. Pittman and UA president Dr. Roger Sayers approached Ficken about assuming the position in a full-time capacity. Although flattered and deeply committed to the college, Ficken was reluctant to take on the deanship. "I was never interested in that level of administration," he said, "even though I had always served an administrative role." One of Ficken's major concerns, which was shared by some of his colleagues, was that he would have a credibility issue as a non-medical doctor running a medical program. Ficken, with a doctorate in medical sociology, was concerned that he would not command respect in this role without a medical degree. Many in the UA administration, including Sayers, did not agree. In Birmingham the administration felt comfortable with Ficken's ability to lead the program. "Birmingham was comfortable because Jim Pittman and I had a good relationship," Ficken said, noting that the animosity that marked the first decade of the college's history had subsided.

A native of Marshall, Oklahoma, Ficken received his baccalaureate degree from Phillips University in Enid, Oklahoma, before going to the University of Kentucky in Lexington. Here Ficken received both a Master's degree (1971) and a Ph.D. (1973) under Dr. Robert Strauss and was exposed to the thinking of William R. Willard, whom he came to admire greatly. It was at Strauss's recommendation and Willard's urging that Ficken joined the CCHS faculty in 1973. "Dr. Ficken was not only a good behavioral scientist, but a very sound citizen who fit very well into the college and gradually developed an excellent program," Willard said of Ficken.[74]

Ficken quickly took on increased responsibilities in the college, serving as director of the office of Medical Student Affairs at two different times while he was chair of the Department of Behavioral Sciences at CCHS in 1977, a post he held for ten years. In 1987 Ficken was appointed associate dean for Academic Affairs, a position he held for almost four years before taking on the deanship.

Ficken was a good choice to lead the college. His tenure in the college gave him an excellent understanding of the program and its history. And with a background in behavioral and community medicine, Ficken valued the goals of the college and what the college meant for Alabama. Likewise, he appreciated the legacy of Bill Willard, who died in 1991 at the age of eighty-three.

"Bill Willard had a major influence on our perspectives and how we did our jobs," said Ficken, noting that he and Harry Knopke used to visit Willard at his home long after the founding dean's retirement. Throughout his tenure, Ficken endeavored to fulfill the goals that his mentor had set for the college, while recognizing the primacy of the educational programs over the outreach efforts.

Challenges in the Residency Program

The 1990s would prove to be a very challenging time for the twenty-year-old residency program. In spite of success in recruiting and the training program itself, a series of administrative changes and other factors left many in the program feeling discouraged.

In 1991 the Department of Family Medicine was headed by Dr. Alan Maxwell, who assumed the position after the departure of Dr. Jerry Jones. Several new faculty members joined the college about this time, all graduates of the residency, including Dr. Robert Ireland (1984), Dr. Jerry McKnight (1985), and Dr. Pam Tietze, (1987). Ireland's background was unusual in that his first career was in the military. A graduate of the U.S. Military Academy at West Point, he had served for five years to repay his military obligation. He then completed medical school in Mississippi and first came to CCHS in the family practice residency. After seven years of private practice he joined the faculty, believing that his experience would be useful to the residents coming behind him. This proved to be the case as his superior clinical skills and his delight in teaching have been recognized repeatedly by the residents.

McKnight, a graduate of the University of Tennessee College of Medicine, joined the college after spending four years fulfilling his National Health Service Corps obligation treating underprivileged patients in a new community health center in eastern Tennessee. "It was very difficult work," he said in an interview, "it was what you'd expect in a place replete with poverty. But, I sort of cut my primary care teeth and [the experience] stood me in good stead coming back [to CCHS in the early 1990s]." McKnight added a high level of clinical skill to the department and later served as chair of family medicine. Pam Tietze completed her residency training in Tuscaloosa because her husband, Paul Tietze, had joined the department in 1985. She shared his interest in family dynamics as an important aspect of family practice.

In 1992 Dr. Elizabeth Philp joined the department. She and her husband, Dr. James Philp, brought expertise in Problem-Based Learning and Objective Structured Clinical Evaluation gained in their service at

Bowman Gray School of Medicine (now Wake Forest University School of Medicine).

Dr. Bobbi Adcock, who completed the residency here in 1991, joined the faculty in 1994 after three years of private practice in Tennessee. An outstanding resident, Dr. Adcock's scholarly interest and commitment to patient care brought needed strengths to the department. At this point the size and strength of the department was at an all-time high, even though medical student interest in primary care was quite low throughout the country. Adcock developed a new teaching clinic at CMC where each medical student would provide continuity of care for one or more patients under her supervision. This was difficult at best because the student on their other clinical rotations would find that the faculty wanted their attention full-time. But continuity of care is one of the major principals of family medicine, and Dr. Adcock's clinic was an innovative attempt to have students experience this aspect of medical practice.

Student interest in family medicine was variable during the nineties. The growth of HMOs and managed care caused a spike in interest at mid-decade as their demand for "gatekeepers" increased. But the gatekeeper concept was soon abandoned, the annual growth rate of managed care companies declined, and the demand for family doctors slowed. In the meantime almost one hundred new residency programs had been established. With a host of new programs available even well-established residencies found recruiting more difficult.

By the middle of the decade, other new faculty members were added. Ficken appointed Dr. Marc Armstrong, who was the first resident here in 1974, to the position of director of the residency program in 1995. Armstrong held this position for four years, during which time he became the medical director of the CMC. Dr. William Owings also joined the college in a full-time capacity at this time. Owings, whose practice in Centreville had been a mainstay of the rural experience for students and residents for thirty years, decided to continue teaching while giving up his responsibilities for his private practice. He was recruited by McKnight and joined the faculty in the family medicine department in 1996.

Enriching Medical Education

Significant changes in the teaching programs for students and residents began in the 1990s. The first of these was the Problem-Based Learning

(PBL) approach to clinical teaching, and the Objective Structured Clinical Evaluation (OSCE) method of evaluating performance. The OSCE methodology fills an often-neglected aspect of medical education—testing the skills of the learner in taking the medical history and performing an appropriate physical examination. Using trained surrogate patients portraying specific diseases, the instructor can observe the learner's performance in the most obvious parts of these procedures and the even more subtle ones. Written and oral tests cannot measure these important parts of clinical practice. Increasingly popular in medical school curricula since the 1970s, PBL and OSCE had caught the attention of former Dean Coggins and Dr. Paul Tietze, an associate professor of family medicine and director of Medical Student Affairs. Coggins and Tietze decided it might prove beneficial for CCHS students and worked together to prepare and submit a grant proposal to the U.S. Department of Health and Human Services; it was funded in 1991. The intent of the program was to incorporate problem-based learning, as the approach is often known, into the clinical clerkships on campus. While these techniques had been applied across the country to the first two years of the medical school curriculum, CCHS was among the first programs to use the method for clinical teaching. This would also prove to serve as excellent preparation for the proposed incorporation of the OSCE into the U.S. Medical Licensure Examination.

The first trial-run OSCE was administered at the CMC in spring 1992. Participating were eighteen third-year medical students, who were asked to rotate through five stations assessing the condition of "patients," volunteers from campus and the community who would act as patients with an assortment of complaints. Students were evaluated on their ability to assess the patient's problem, perform an appropriate physical examination, diagnose the condition, and communicate with the patient.

The second OSCE was a much larger effort administered one year later under the leadership of Dr. Elizabeth Philp. She was appointed as the director of OSCE at CCHS. She strongly believed in the value of the PBL/OSCE method. "Medical education had too often deteriorated to multiple choice questions which taught and tested knowledge, but not clinical ability to relate to patients," said Philp.[75]

Under her leadership, and with support from Dr. Harold Fallon, the dean of UASOM who replaced Pittman in 1993, the OSCE was given to third-year medical students from both the Huntsville and Tuscaloosa campuses in May 1993. Clinical faculty from all three UASOM campuses participated in the evaluation process in Tuscaloosa. This marked the first time that medical students from the entire class and faculty from all three campuses joined together for a clinical teaching exercise in Tuscaloosa.

One reason for bringing the entire student body to Tuscaloosa, along with faculty members from Birmingham and Huntsville, was a matter of space. Logistically, performing an OSCE is very demanding of space, equipment, and faculty and staff time. It was logical to do the early annual exercises in Tuscaloosa, but Dean Fallon's decision to do so meant more than that. Even relatively new CCHS faculty members knew that the integrity of the medical school program had been threatened as recently as 1990. It was a demonstration of support for CCHS by Dean Fallon. He was also helpful to Ficken in the negotiation with DCH for increased support for the college. He strongly supported John Wheat's development of the Rural Health and Rural Medical Scholars Programs.

The OSCE program received rave reviews from all of those involved. Comments by some of the examinees described the process as "excellent," "helpful and very well executed," and as a "good learning experience." As a result, students at the Birmingham campus were required to participate in 1994.

By 1995 the UASOM Medical Education Committee approved the requirement that all students pass the OSCE before graduation, beginning with the graduating class of 1997. The OSCE was to be given after the usual completion of the junior year to allow for remediation of any areas where a student's performance may have been inadequate.

During the late 1990s, OSCE was incorporated into other areas of teaching at UASOM, thus speaking to the effectiveness of this approach. On the Birmingham campus, for example, as an introductory course in medicine was developed for first- and second-year students, the faculty there worked with Elizabeth Philp to develop "mini-OSCEs" for use in test blocks throughout the course.

Teaching Clinical Pharmacy

The rapid growth in the number and variety of new drugs created a new challenge for clinical teaching and prescribing of medications. In 1992 faculty in internal medicine and family medicine joined with the School of Pharmacy at Auburn University to bring clinical pharmacists into full-time positions in the college. An initial shared position between the two departments soon led to a full-time position in each department. The rapid acceptance of pharmacists by medical students, residents, and their attending physicians testified to their usefulness as members of the clinical team. In the late 1990s a third position was developed for a pharmacist to participate in the rural program. The pharmacists participate in hospital rounds, in the clinic, in didactic sessions, and in offering short electives for the residents and medical students. This is one vivid example of the team approach to clinical teaching and patient care that has proved to be successful.

A New Dean for UASOM

Dean Fallon would prove to be supportive of such innovative efforts during his four-year tenure as dean of UASOM. A graduate of Yale University School of Medicine, he completed his residency in internal medicine at the University of North Carolina, School of Medicine. He then returned to Yale where he conducted research on disease of the liver. After a one-year stint at the University of Utrecht, Netherlands, Fallon joined the faculty at the University of North Carolina, School of Medicine, Chapel Hill, where he distinguished himself in research and patient care in gastroenterology. In 1974 he became the chair of the Department of Medicine, Medical College of Virginia, Virginia Commonwealth University, in Richmond, where he remained until 1993 when he left to become dean at UASOM.

Making Strides in Community Medicine

One of the distinguishing features of the CCHS program was its unique emphasis on community medicine and rural health. Dean Willard had viewed this as the backbone of the program, believing that a focus on this overlooked area of medical education would help sensitize future physicians to the various social, emotional, and environmental factors influencing the health of a patient and his or her family. In the 1990s this thinking was still very much a part of the belief system of the college, yet for various reasons the medical student curriculum included very little exposure to community medicine; in 1992 the required rotation in this area was only two weeks of the six-week rotation in family medicine. This was quite a decrease in rotation length from the program that was begun in the 1970s with an intensive two-month rotation in community medicine. Dr. James Leeper, chair of the Department of Community and Behavioral Medicine since 1987, noted in an interview, "we were hanging on by the skin of our teeth."

That was soon to change, however; in 1993 the community medicine experience became required for all UASOM students. This was largely due to the influence of the Alabama Family Practice Rural Health Board, which was formed in 1990 by an act of the legislature to tackle the problem of insufficient distribution of family physicians in the state, particularly in rural areas. The eleven-member board, which included CCHS residency graduates Dr. Sandral Hullett and Dr. Michael McBrearty, encouraged UASOM to help address the problem, and a rotation in rural medicine was created with funds from the board. At that time students from all three UASOM campuses started a four-week rural medicine experience in the third year. This had a positive effect on the department, according to Leeper. "It stabilized the situation for the first time, the first time the whole system bought into it," he said.

A key contributor during this time was a new faculty member in the department, Dr. John Wheat, who accepted a joint appointment in the departments of Behavioral and Community Medicine and Internal Medicine in 1990. A native of Alabama, Wheat received his medical degree from UASOM, completed his internal medicine training in the U.S. Navy and the Mayo Graduate School of Medicine, and his M.P.H. from the University of North Carolina. He was hired to help develop the rural medicine mission of CCHS, a task he assumed with enthusiasm. In the years that followed, he drew on his training at Chapel Hill in health policy and administration, helping the college to form critical partnerships with key individuals and organizations to help enhance the concept of community medicine.

One of the key initiatives undertaken in CCHS during this time was a deliberate attempt to strengthen the rural medical pipeline. Through establishment of a series of programs designed to find and nurture students from rural areas, the intent was—and is—to recruit medical students who will seek to practice in underserved areas. The program has been conducted in partnership with UA, UASOM, the Alabama Department of Public Health, and the Alabama Family Practice Rural Health

Board. Two key aspects of the rural medical pipeline were the Rural Health Scholars program and the Rural Medical Scholars program.

The Rural Health Scholars Program was founded in 1993 by Wheat to address promising high school juniors from rural areas and introduce them to college life. Through university courses, special seminars, workshops, and activities, the students were exposed to college life while learning more about health and medical careers in rural areas.

The success of the program led to the establishment of another in 1996, the Rural Medical Scholars Program. This concept involves a five-year track of medical studies, including a year prior to entry in medical school. College seniors or graduate students from rural areas are chosen to participate in this highly selective program each year. Rural Medical Scholars focuses on primary care, community medicine and rural medicine practice, with an eye toward ultimately increasing the number of doctors who choose to practice in the rural areas of the state.

Hard Times

Unfortunately, even with such visible successes occurring in the college, CCHS struggled financially through much of Ficken's deanship. In January 1991 Governor Guy Hunt ordered a 3.7 percent across-the-board cutback of the state budget, which had an immediate impact on the budget of the university. The economic slowdown affecting the nation had hit Alabama hard, and the state's tax revenues had come up short. The university—and ultimately CCHS—lost hundreds of thousands of dollars in state revenue. Like the leaders before him, Ficken would learn early in his career as dean the challenges associated with running the program on a limited budget that was often reduced in the middle of a budgetary year. Working to accomplish the goals of the college was frustrating under such circumstances, but it was not the last time that CCHS would see its funding reduced.

"Proration," Ficken would later reflect, "is a thorn in the side of all of the divisions on this campus . . . and all have suffered because of it."[76]

It was later that year that UA administrators made a decision to do something to shore up the programs in the university in the face of serious declines in state funding. Years of reduced appropriations from the state had taken a toll on the goals of the university and there was concern about the effect that these shortfalls would have on the quality of the university's academic programs. In response, in May 1992 President Sayers announced a capital campaign with a goal of $165 million. The goal of the five-year campaign was to augment new academic areas and strengthen programs, not to replace state funds that everyone hoped would be reinstated at some point in the future. The private support garnered by the campaign was designed to raise much-needed funds for endowing academic programs, chairs, professorships, scholarships, and even new facilities. CCHS was asked to be part of the effort and the goal of the college was set at $6 million. Dr. Arthur "Pete" Snyder of the CCHS Department of Surgery was asked to chair the steering committee for the CCHS campaign; he was assisted by thirteen others in the college.

In the in-house newsletter, Ficken addressed the reasoning behind the campaign and his wish that the faculty and alumni would do their part: "As you know, state funds are not the reliable resource they were in the past and they have never been available at a level that would allow us to successfully pursue all of our goals. To preserve this success and to assure the future, we must now develop private resources," he wrote, going on to stress the need for scholarships for rural students and funds for strengthening the CCHS faculty.[77]

The campaign was an enormous undertaking for the college, reflected Ficken. "Very few of the deans had any experience in this sort of thing," he said. "It was something we really had to gear up for." Ficken and several others on campus attended a training session designed to teach the fundamentals of this major type of fundraising.

The campaign went very well, bringing in more than $200 million to the university. One excellent outcome of the campaign for CCHS was a $1 million gift to the college to endow a chair in family medicine. Mrs. Celia Wallace, chief executive officer of Springhill Memorial Hospital in Mobile, pledged the funds in 1994 in memory of her late husband, Dr. Gerald Leon Wallace. Dr. Wallace, who founded the Springhill Hospital in 1974, was a firm believer in the importance of primary care and the importance of the community hospital. In acknowledging the generous gift, Ficken noted that both Mrs. Wallace and CCHS appreciated the value and importance of providing high-caliber training to family physicians. The Gerald Leon Wallace Endowed Chair in Family Medicine was the first endowed chair in the college and one of the first endowed chairs of family medicine in the country. It was a fitting gift for one of the most productive family practice residencies in the Southeast.

The Lister Hill Society

In 1995 the leaders of the college took another step toward bolstering its tenuous financial situation by reviving the Lister Hill Society. This fundraising organization, developed in 1975 to support CCHS and help advance the field of family medicine, had long been an important source of private support. These funds had been used to underwrite new initiatives in the college, purchase new equipment, and strengthen established programs. Members of the Lister Hill Society had also served an important steering function for the college by providing evaluations of current programs and helping to anticipate and provide for future needs.

Although CCHS had been well served by the works of the society, college leaders had allowed the organization to languish. In 1994 a decision was made to reactivate the group. Under the leadership of Dr. Lorin Baumhover, director of the CCHS Center for the Study of Aging, efforts to add to the membership of the society and solicit more funding for the college were stepped up and slowly the organization—and its usefulness to CCHS—grew. With support from the chancellor's office and from Mr. Jack Warner, chairman of the board for Tuscaloosa-based Gulf States Paper Company, an annual fund raiser was started. From 1995 to 1998 under the leadership of Dr. William Winternitz and Dr. Wilmer Coggins, contributions to the organization quadrupled. This money was used to fund scholarships, publish an alumni newsletter, support student and resident travel to national meetings, and provide start-up funds for research projects.

Strengthening Ties with DCH

The financial constraints put on the college in the form of reduced state appropriations took a toll once more in 1993 when the university budget was prorated again. CCHS was especially hard hit during this time: its budget was reduced by 5.03 percent—$200,000—far more than any other colleges proportionally. College administrators were especially frustrated by the size of the reduction to CCHS; the only other college on campus to see such a large cut was the College of Engineering, which was prorated at 2.5 percent, only one half of the amount at which CCHS was assessed. Ficken pointed out that this was one of the disadvantages of having a clinical services foundation that provided additional funds for operating the college and also demonstrated "the level of priority this college held in the scheme of things on this campus."[78]

When the university budgets were cut again in 1995, the cuts resulted in the reduction of eight staff and faculty positions in CCHS, the first time such a measure had to be taken in the history of the college. "It was a very tough time," recalled Ficken.

The continual decline of the college's funding was watched with consternation. It was noted that in 1993, approximately 40 percent of the college's support came from state funds and by 1994, state support provided only 37 percent of the college's budget. This was not expected to improve in the foreseeable future. The program, CCHS administrators noted, was merely "state assisted," but not state supported. Fears that funding shortfalls would necessitate cuts in the residency program led to a decision to ask DCH for more support.

By the mid-1990s DCH had become a regional medical center with more than five hundred beds and had been expanded to include the Northport Medical Center, adjacent to Tuscaloosa, and Fayette Hospital in Fayette County. Renamed the DCH Regional Medical System, the hospital had formed an important partnership with the university that spanned more than twenty years. The collaboration allowed for the delivery of critical inpatient and outpatient services to west Alabama's citizens, including the area's indigent.

Negotiations began in spring 1993 with the DCH leadership, including Mr. Samuel Phelps, chairman of the board for DCH, Mr. James H. Ford, Jr., DCH chief administrator, President Sayers, and Mr. Sam Faucett, a local businessman and trustee for both DCH and the Capstone Health Services Foundation. Representing CCHS were Dean Ficken and Dr. John Durant, senior vice president for Health Affairs at UAB, who had agreed to support the negotiations. Ficken described Durant as a "good friend" to CCHS and instrumental in helping to get DCH to recognize its responsibilities for the educational programs that provided many beneficial services to the hospital. Because Ficken and his staff had forged good relations with the administrators at DCH, there was optimism that DCH would agree to increase its support in this time of need.

The contributions of DCH to the college were not in question: the growing community-based hospital had made the residency program possible, and the 190 residents that received their training there to date were well prepared for careers in medicine. Since 1982, when the hospital made its first direct financial contribution to the program, support to the program totaled $2.7 million. By 1992–93, DCH was contributing $560,000 annually to the CCHS educational programs; the bulk of this sum went toward paying the stipends of the thirty-six residents in the CCHS family practice residency, over a third of its annual cost.

But the educational programs at the college made significant contributions to the hospital, too. CCHS faculty and residents provided a great deal of care in the hospital services for children, as well as for obstetrical and internal medicine patients. A great deal of this was charity care in the tradition of teaching hospitals. Through its weekly series of noon conferences CCHS also provided most of the continuing medical education to the doctors and other health care professionals in the community, the education that is required for continued licensure for doctors. Authorized by the Accreditation Council for Continuing Medical Education through the UASOM, the college provided valuable CME credits to those who needed them, thus helping health care professionals meet their requirements while elevating the care standards in the community. Each year more than one hundred CME programs were offered by the college, and as many as three thousand hours of CME credit were earned by local physicians, pharmacists, nurses, and social workers. Documentation of attendance for participants, as well as the planning and funding of programs, was an expense borne by the college.

CCHS also provided an excellent health sciences library for the use of the medical and nursing staff. At that time every hospital was required to have a library, as mandated by the Joint Commission on Accreditation of Hospitals (now known as the Joint Commission on Accreditation of Healthcare Organizations). The library, located in the Education Tower, helped the hospital fulfill this requirement without having to maintain a library of its own. By 1990 the library's holdings had grown to 10,000 monographs, 10,000 bound journal volumes, 475 serial subscriptions, and thousands of audiovisual items with an emphasis on primary care and clinical medicine.

CCHS also provided another very real benefit to DCH in the form of income. Because of the hospital's participation in the UASOM graduate medical education program, it was able to receive payment from Medicare for both direct and indirect costs of the educational program for residents, support that equaled more than $2.2 million in 1992–93 alone. The following year, that number was increased to more than $2.5 million.

Of this, only $560,000 was passed on to CCHS, a sum that equaled only 6.8 percent of the college's total budget. CCHS administrators pointed out that many other community hospitals provided much greater financial support of their residency programs. In a survey of similar programs in community hospitals in the U.S., hospital support for their residency programs ranged from 20 to 36 percent of the cost of the program.

Negotiations between the two organizations resulted in an increase to CCHS of $140,000, but Ficken hoped the hospital would be able to do more. In 1995 the college again faced additional cuts: the total loss of state income to the college due to proration amounted to more than $736,000 over just a few years. CCHS administrators appealed to the hospital to do more, requesting $1.4 million, half of the hospital's income, for the two medical education programs. However, the hospital was facing its own financial difficulties due to reduced revenues, in addition to a looming threat by the government to cut Medicare and Medicaid funding to hospitals. The result, warned DCH administrator Ford, "does not bode well for medical education."[79]

In an editorial in the local newspaper, Ficken talked about the disastrous effect that funding shortfalls would have on the medical education program, and ultimately on health care in Alabama. In it he addressed the productivity of the program: since 1974, 210 family physicians had received their training in Tuscaloosa. Of those, 108 were practicing in Alabama. Important work was also being done at the CMC, where many of the area's medically indigent received their care. As a result of the services provided by CCHS faculty and residents in 1994, the clinic provided more than $2 million in nonreimbursed medical care. "This is by any standard a gift to the healthcare of the community," wrote Ficken.[80] He went on to note that the School of Medicine and DCH were working together to solve the funding problems but that the future of the program was uncertain.

Indeed, in north Alabama a similar scenario was being played out. In 1995 faced with slashed budgets, administrators at the School of Primary Medical Care at UA-Huntsville announced its closing. Like CCHS, the school was faced with high budget cuts under Governor Fob James that threatened its future. In May 1995 the president of UAH, Dr. Frank A. Franz, announced that the medical program there would close in order that the university could focus on its primary and most "strategically im-

A SPECIAL KIND OF DOCTOR
A History of the College of Community Health Sciences
Patricia J. West with Wilmer J. Coggins, M.D.
ADDENDUM
(insert on page 115 before subhead)

Obstetrics – Gynecology Fellowship

One of the greatest health care needs in rural Alabama has been and continues to be better obstetrical care. Although substantial numbers of family practice residents had established practices in rural areas, too few of them included obstetrics. The training program, under the direction of Dr. Paul Mozley, was well set up to provide a sound program in obstetrical care. DCH Regional Medical Center had a very active obstetrical service and Dr. Mozley, and his faculty were highly motivated to teach the residents. Unlike many family medicine programs there were no residents in obstetrics to compete for patients. In rural areas of Alabama, there were virtually no specialists in OB/Gyn to compete with the family doctors who might practice obstetrics. One disincentive was that larger towns and small city hospitals were not inclined to offer obstetrical privileges to family doctors if there were obstetricians on their staff, although older family doctors who had established obstetrical practices might continue their practices until retirement.

Yet another barrier for the residents was the high ratio of women with potential high-risk elements in their pregnancies, such as anemia, malnutrition, primary hypertension and diabetes. Many of the residents who might have chosen to provide obstetrical services to potential mothers who were at less risk did not feel well equipped to handle these more complex patients. Several rural areas in Alabama had no nearby hospitals providing obstetrical services for those who might require referral.

With this background, Dr. Mozley and his faculty developed a one-year fellowship, primarily for residents in the Tuscaloosa program. There would be one fellowship offered each year. If none of the Capstone residents applied, the position could be filled by a resident from another program.

Financial assistance, principally to provide a stipend for the fellow, was awarded by the Alabama Family Practice Rural Health Board.

The first fellow chosen was Dr. Cindy Dedmon. After the fellowship year she joined the College's Department of Obstetrics and Gynecology to encourage other residents to follow in her footsteps and to participate in teaching medical students and residents in their required obstetrical rotations. Nine fellows have since participated in the one-year experience, and eight of them are now practicing in small towns. One, Dr. Melissa Behringer, is a faculty member in the CCHS "sister" program, the branch campus at the University of Alabama School of Medicine in Huntsville.

Although these numbers may seem small, each of these young physicians provide a vital service to women who live in areas with poor access to obstetrical services and who have limited access to long distance transportation when labor begins. In our documented experience, the infant mortality rate in Pickens County, Alabama declined from 17.8 per thousand in 1986 to 6.9 per thousand in 1991. This compares favorably to the national rate of 6.8 per thousand in 1991.

portant" missions of high-technology research and education, including science, engineering, mathematics, computer science, and other associated fields.

Concern about the closure of the program ran high among medical groups in the state. According to the Alabama Chapter of the American Academy of Family Physicians, sixty of the state's sixty-seven counties had recently been designated as "health professions shortage areas" by the federal government; members of the academy believed the loss of the Huntsville program would hamper the state's ability to produce needed primary care doctors. Ultimately, UAB announced its decision to assume control of the Huntsville program in order to keep the school from being closed; today UAB continues to operate the program as an entity that is completely separate from UAH. But the possibility of losing the program caused alarm in Tuscaloosa, fearing that CCHS would face a similar crisis in the coming years. In a letter to Mr. Bryan Kindred, chief operating officer at DCH, Dr. Gary Magouirk, the president of the Alabama Chapter of the American Academy of Family Physicians, and Dr. John Brandon, who was active in the same organization, addressed the general state of concern that many felt when the president of UAH made his announcement. Magouirk and Brandon were former residents at CCHS, and both had become prominent in state medical issues.

"Upon learning of the past problems with inadequate funding from DCH Health Care Authority to the College of Community Health Sciences . . . , our members could foresee significant potential for this situation to be duplicated in Tuscaloosa within the coming year," they wrote.[81]

By 1996 support from DCH to CCHS topped the $1 million mark, and a crisis was averted.

Success at the Capstone

In spite of the external forces that threatened to hold back the college, growth was seen on several fronts. At the CMC, for example, the mid-nineties were boom years. The small, ambulatory clinic that started in a small house on Sixth Avenue was becoming a major force in health care delivery in the area. During a ten-year period from 1984–94, the number of patients served at the Capstone nearly doubled. In 1983 more than

8,500 patients made 27,320 visit to the clinic. By 1990 more than 11,600 patients made almost 64,500 office visits. In 1993 the number of patients had risen to more than 13,800; they made almost 70,000 office visits.

The services provided by the CMC were also expanding: various support groups had been set up, such as one for patients with diabetes and one for patients with severe premenstrual syndrome (PMS). A new statewide effort called the MediKids program enabled the pediatrics faculty to expand its services in screening and preventive programs for children. The faculties in family medicine and internal medicine also expanded the clinic's occupational health services, which had been established in the 1980s during Coggins's tenure as dean. In late 1994 the college secured contracts with the Harrison Division of General Motors and Kansas City–Southern Railroad in Tuscaloosa to provide such services as assistance with meeting the requirements of the Occupational Health and Safety Act (OSHA). In the mid-1990s the college started the Physicians Access Line or PAL, a regional twenty-four-hour patient referral network. The program, made possible through an agreement with the Rural Alabama Health Alliance (RAHA), was designed to give area doctors, particularly those in rural areas, a way to follow their patients who were referred for specialized care. Another area that CMC would move into by 1998 was the offering of social services for patients. Through a joint program with the School of Social Work, a full-time social worker was added to the staff at the CMC. The program was growing to meet the needs of the community, and the faculty and administration of the College could be proud of the gains that were being made.

Changing Leadership

In July 1996 Dean Ficken opted to take early retirement and leave the university after nearly twenty-three years. The many incentives offered by the university, combined with a desire to spend more time with his grandchildren and increase his commitment to his church, prompted the decision. Although he would remain active in the college, especially in the area of fundraising, Ficken felt it was time to move on.

Dr. Michael McBrearty, a family practitioner in Fairhope, Alabama, who completed the family practice residency in the 1970s, spoke about the contributions that Ficken made. "Dr. Scutchfield was the chair of the new family medicine/community medicine program, but Roland was the one who really helped define what community medicine meant," said McBrearty.[82] McBrearty also spoke of Ficken's considerate nature and outstanding support of individuals and the program. "There has never been a time that he has not been an advocate for the mission of CCHS, and I think his own experience has helped him convey the importance of that mission,"[83] McBrearty said.

The major challenge the college then faced was trying to identify a person to assume the deanship on a temporary basis until a new dean could be identified. UASOM dean Dr. Harold Fallon and Dr. Robert Centor, associate dean for Primary Care at UASOM, had stepped in to help after Ficken's retirement. In August 1996, Fallon asked Centor to serve as interim dean while a search was conducted. Centor agreed to be in Tuscaloosa two days each week as interim dean.

Centor would ultimately spend almost two years in this position. As a primary care physician and a native of a small town in Virginia, he had a feeling for small towns and a dedication to primary care. Centor was educated in Virginia, earning his B.A. from the University of Virginia in 1971 and an M.D. from the Medical College of Virginia in 1975, where he later served as chief medical resident. Centor then joined the faculty of Medical College of Virginia, where he eventually served as professor and chairman of general internal medicine. While in Virginia he served as the director of internal medicine education at St. Mary's Hospital in Richmond for three years. He joined UASOM in 1993 where he served as the director of the general internal medicine program. He quickly distinguished himself as an outstanding clinical teacher and has been recognized for excellence in teaching medical students many times over the past eight years. Because of his interest in teaching, he had been instrumental in encouraging selected members of the UASOM faculty to upgrade their clinical teaching skills.

One of Centor's responsibilities during his tenure would be to refine and focus the mission of the College in concert with the new leadership at UA, Dr. Andrew Sorensen, who assumed the post of president after Sayers retired, and Dr. Nancy Barrett, the university's new provost. Both were enthusiastic about helping to steer CCHS into the future. Sorensen in particular, who held both a master's and doctoral degree in medical sociology, had an academic appointment in Behavioral and Community Medicine in CCHS and would prove to be supportive of the college.

Another priority for Centor was improving the finances of the college.

Although Ficken had successfully worked with DCH to increase their support, years of proration and a lack of clinical income still hurt the college. Centor made the difficult decision to increase the clinical income from the CMC, a valuable source of revenue to any medical school. To do this, Centor revamped the rewards system of the Capstone Health Services Foundation. Prior to this time, faculty salary supplements were paid from the foundation based on volume as well as income generated. Under Centor's direction, the system was changed to supplements based on generated income alone, a move that he believed would increase productivity. Although this decision to alter the salary plan was controversial and unpopular with some in the college, administrators believed it had to be done.

"I knew I was going to have to aggravate some people and make some people unhappy, but I knew I was going to have to do that if CCHS was going to survive," said Centor in a recent interview. "The program was under a lot of financial stress at that point."

Dr. Marc Armstrong, associate dean for Clinical Affairs, agreed with the decision. "We were in a world of hurt economically and he [Centor] approved a plan to fix it and supported me and John Maxwell [administrator of the CMC] in instituting it," said Armstrong. "Dr. Centor said, 'yes, we will have the salary plan and it will be based on productivity, not on academic rank; your state salary is through academic rank and scholarly research, and your foundation salary is through your productivity in patient care.'" These changes would demand more time and effort from the faculty and several faculty members would leave as a result of these changes. However, the finances of the college were undoubtedly strengthened during Centor's term as interim dean: income to the program increased almost 50 percent during Centor's first year in Tuscaloosa.

The Press for More Space

Centor saw another need as he served at CCHS and that was for additional, modernized space. When he assumed the post in 1996, the college had grown to thirty-five full-time faculty, forty-six part-time faculty, and ninety-five staff members, including the nursing staff at CMC. By the twenty-second year of the residency, 222 residents had completed the program and almost 350 medical students had finished their clinical training at CCHS. The program was growing, but the facilities needed to accommodate them were not. Everyone involved in the program recognized that, as a result, the quality of the program suffered.

It was a 1996 evaluation by the Residency Review Committee of Family Medicine Programs, the accreditation body for residency programs, that highlighted the inadequacy of the facilities. By 1996 the faculty and staff of the college were spread out in five locations in four different buildings, hampering communication and productivity. "It was pretty clear that having the administration two miles away from the clinic and across the street from the hospital was pretty dysfunctional," said Centor.

A new building would also attract residents to the program, administrators believed. As medical student interest in family medicine nationwide had waned, so had the number of applications for the residency. CCHS administrators believed a new building to replace the CMC was a necessity. "We would be competitive with the other residencies that were opening, all of whom had new buildings. [A new facility] could be wired for the twenty-first century through the Internet and . . . [we could have] electronic medical records and . . . it [would] be designed for the efficient delivery of outpatient care," Armstrong said in a recent interview.

Appeals to UA administrators for new facilities began with Sorensen in 1996. Although CCHS was on the list for capital improvements, conversations with the university administration indicated that a lack of money made a new building a distant possibility. The bottom line was that if the college needed a new building its leaders would have to raise the money themselves.

In 1997 Barrett, in her role as provost, convened a committee to review the possibility of combining all health-related activities, including the departments of nursing, social work, student health, speech and hearing, and CCHS. After several meetings, the idea was dismissed because the cost associated with building such a large facility made it unrealistic.

Efforts to raise the funds needed to build a new clinic began at once with the support of Sorensen, who also agreed to request an educational bond issue for a significant portion of the costs. The Health Services Foundation also agreed to underwrite a portion of the bond payments. Planning for the new building was initiated by Mr. John Maxwell, administrator of the CMC. He worked up cost estimates and planned the new, efficient space.

In the meantime, other improvements to the program were being made. Sorenson offered to provide the college with $400,000 to upgrade the computer systems for the college, which had few computers available for research, teaching, patient care, or even communication between the widely dispersed faculty and staff. Under the direction of Dr. McHattie of OB/GYN, followed by Dr. Michael Taylor, who joined the Department of Pediatrics in 1991, the plans for a major upgrade in computer-based systems would encompass virtually all areas of the college—even several multimedia classrooms were to be installed. "Dr. Fallon and Dr. Centor were very interested in trying to improve our technology," said Taylor in an interview.

He viewed the addition of these facilities as being indispensable in teaching the next generation of physicians. Indeed, many of the advances made in the program, and to the program, began to have an impact. The results would soon be felt throughout the college as it entered the next phase in its history.

The Renascence of CCHS

The twenty-fifth anniversary for CCHS in 1997 went by with little fanfare. The celebratory activities that might ordinarily mark such an event were tempered by two major changes in leadership in the university system in Birmingham and in Tuscaloosa. In both places the changes would bode well for CCHS.

In Birmingham Harold Fallon retired from the deanship at UASOM, to be succeeded by William Deal. Dr. Fallon had been supportive to the concepts and efforts of CCHS, and had urged them to begin some efforts in clinical research. He also helped the college in its negotiations with DCH for increased support.

The new dean, Dr. William B. Deal, was first appointed on an interim basis. Deal had been in Birmingham since 1991, when he was appointed by Dean Pittman to act as senior associate dean of UASOM. Educated at the University of North Carolina, Deal received his postgraduate training in internal medicine and infectious diseases at the University of Florida Hospital. He later joined the faculty at the University of Florida and moved through the ranks to become associate dean and then dean. Deal was named dean of UASOM in November 1997 and would prove to be a strong supporter of the work being done at CCHS.

Deal was familiar with CCHS. He had been head of the LCME accreditation site visit team for UASOM in 1990. He noted then that there was insufficient communication between UASOM and the branch campuses. He noted that not enough attention was being paid to the branch campuses and early in his role as associate dean, he made a point of visiting each campus. To many, this opened the door to more cooperative relations between UASOM and the programs in Tuscaloosa and Huntsville.

In Tuscaloosa, Centor continued to act as interim dean of CCHS. Yet in spite of Centor's effectiveness and his administrative expertise, his part-time status on the Tuscaloosa campus frustrated many at CCHS who felt that the campus needed a full-time senior administrator. The CCHS faculty wanted the college to secure a permanent person who could guide the program into the future. UA President Andrew Sorensen, well aware of the disadvantages of such an arrangement, was actively involved in the search for a new dean.

During this period, Centor was able to recruit one individual who soon became recognized as important to the future of the program: Dr. William Curry. A general internist from Carrollton in Pickens County, Alabama, Curry had ties to CCHS and the university that extended back many years. Appointed by Deal to serve as associate dean for Clinical Affairs at CCHS and assistant dean for Rural Medicine for the entire medical school, Curry would play a key role in redefining the rural mission of the college.

"My legacy as interim dean will be the successful recruitment of Bill Curry," said Centor at the time of Curry's appointment.[84] Convinced of Curry's leadership ability, Centor worked hard to bring him to CCHS.

Curry received his baccalaureate degree from UA and his medical degree from Vanderbilt University. After medical school he completed a residency in internal medicine and then returned to his home town Carrollton, in Pickens County to practice medicine in order to fulfill an obligation to the National Health Service Corps. This federal program, which is administered by the U.S. Department of Health and Human Services, offers educational scholarships for aspiring health care professionals who agree, in turn, to commit to practice in medically underserved areas. Pickens County, Alabama, was one such area. Curry soon discovered he loved serving his community in this way. After his two-year service commitment, Curry returned to Vanderbilt to complete a fourth-year residency, serving as chief resident from 1981–82. At the end of his postgraduate training, Curry was offered a faculty position at Vanderbilt, but he instead opted to return to Carrollton to practice.

Curry had discovered that he thrived on the challenge of serving his rural patients. "People told me I'd be wasting what I had learned," he said in an interview, "but I found just the opposite to be true."[85] He noted that he used everything he had been taught and was constantly expanding his knowledge to keep pace with the needs of his patients. During his time in Carrollton, Curry also had other experiences that would serve him well in his capacity as dean. Like many rural hospitals, Pickens County Medical Center in Carrollton was in serious financial difficulty during the 1980s. Curry and his colleagues offered to serve on the management board of the hospital, believing that they could provide direction to the administration for more efficient operation of the hospital. Their guidance helped to stabilize the hospital's tenuous financial situation, and their intimate knowledge and support of the hospital helped to attract new physicians to the community.

But in spite of the satisfaction he gained from private practice, Curry wished to teach, and he accepted a position offered by Winternitz to serve as an adjunct faculty member in the Department of Internal Medicine in 1979, a position he held for almost twenty years. In this capacity he served as an attending physician for the college's inpatient service at DCH periodically throughout the years, a commitment that meant remaining in Tuscaloosa overnight while maintaining his practice in Carrollton. Curry also supervised the numerous residents and students who chose his practice for their rural health experience.

Curry had served in a leadership capacity for several professional organizations, including the presidency of the Alabama Society of Internal Medicine, the presidency of the Medical Association of the State of Alabama, and the chair of the medical association's ad hoc committee on rural medicine and physician supply to rural areas. This effort led to new state laws expanding the medical scholarship program, as well as expansion of the role of nurse practitioners and physicians' assistants. As an advocate of rural medicine and its importance, Curry also helped to organize the Rural Alabama Health Alliance in the early 1990s.

In addition to the important function that Curry would have in managing the clinical affairs of the college and the other larger roles that he would come to play in the development of the college, his appointment in June 1997 as assistant dean for Rural Programs for the entire UASOM had added significance. It was with this appointment by Deal that CCHS was recognized as the rural health campus for the entire medical school, an affirmation of the work that was being done in Tuscaloosa to train doctors for careers in rural areas. Deal noted in an interview that rural medicine "should be Tuscaloosa's," noting that CCHS could "do this better than anybody else in the state."

Much of the credit for the wide recognition that the college received for its commitment to rural medical education must be given to the work of Dr. James Leeper as chair of the Department of Behavioral and Community Medicine and Dr. John Wheat as director of the Rural Health Scholars and Rural Medical Scholars programs. Their efforts in the community medicine aspect of the college were burgeoning. In particular, the attention being paid to the development of the "medical pipeline" was starting to pay dividends: the programs were attracting top-notch students and were receiving wide recognition in the state. It was a signal development in the history of the college.

New Leadership

In late 1997 Curry was asked to serve as the next dean of CCHS, effective in July 1998. His leadership skills and his ability to unite people as a team were contributing factors. In his first joint meeting of the faculty and staff, Curry outlined his initiatives for the college. His goals included the development of the long-hoped-for new building that would house all the personnel and activities of the college together. He also expressed a desire to expand and improve the clinical program in this new space, to improve the services to the patients of the clinic. He also spoke of the need for faculty and staff development, both in terms of research as well as teaching skills. Lastly, he emphasized the need for major upgrades to the information technology in the college. One of the centerpieces of this initiative would be a new management information system, but he also envisioned new networking capabilities and an electronic medical-records system for use at the CMC. In his presentation Curry spoke gratefully of the dedication of the faculty and staff of the college, as well as their loyalty, skills, and openness to new methods and technology. He was counting on these qualities as he implemented his plan to improve the college.

Numerous challenges faced Curry as he assumed the deanship. Although multiple improvements had been made to the program in recent years, more needed to be done. The financial condition of the college was still insufficient to support the ambitious new goals. A severe lack of technological capabilities, such as up-to-date computer equipment, also handicapped the program and its faculty. Likewise, the family practice residency, long the centerpiece of the program, was in danger of losing its accreditation due to the inadequacy of the physical plant at the CMC.

In order to address financial concerns within the college, Curry immediately instituted the means by which the college could better organize, track, and ultimately boost its fund raising efforts. Dean Curry established the Office of Advancement in the college in 1999 to be headed by longtime staff member Mrs. Vicki Johnson. The office was designed to provide a central place from which gifts to the college could be solicited and managed.

Replacement of the CMC was also an urgent need, and Dean Curry immediately set out to secure the new building. To help with the effort, Curry appointed Dr. Marc Armstrong, who then served as the medical director of the clinic, as the lead person in planning the new clinical facility. Although progress had been made on the planning for a new clinic, its construction was not yet guaranteed. Critical questions related to funding, location, and design still had to be answered. Yet with the future of the residency program literally resting on the construction of a new facility, the administration could not afford to delay. Armstrong, together with clinic administrator John Maxwell, pushed the university to help make the building a reality, and several months later, under the leadership of the new dean, the college had a preliminary set of architectural plans for the new facility in hand and approval from the university board of trustees to proceed.

While work continued on obtaining a new facility, a concerted effort was made to upgrade the college, including the CMC, by way of information technology. One of the first areas of interest was upgrading the computer capabilities of CCHS while improving the technical skills of the faculty. This was deemed to be an important step for meeting the demands of modern medical practice and improving communication among the faculty and staff who worked in widely separated buildings. A key step in instituting such changes was a decision to name Dr. Michael Taylor as assistant to the dean for medical information. This position had previously been held by Dr. Thomas McHattie, an obstetrician who left CCHS in 2001. Taylor had led several initiatives in the area of technology upgrade and in this new capacity, he would be able to do even more. New initiatives included the introduction of computer instruction into the student rotations. Likewise, students began receiving instruction from Mrs. Nelle Williams, interim director of the Health Sciences Library, on the use of computer-based research tools such as MD Consult, continuing the long tradition in CCHS of teaching students in computer-based research.

The need to upgrade the computers and computer systems remained paramount: students needed new skills in searching for the ever-expanding journals, medical texts, and Web sites that provide contemporary medical information, and the equipment available to them was inadequate. The upgrading of the college computer lab had become a high priority. In 1999 the college was also able to make a major upgrade to its computer facilities for students through the generosity of Drs. William and James Shamblin.

In August of that year, Taylor had approached the Lister Hill Society for funds for upgrading the computer systems for the students. "I had started the process of asking various people about getting the money and then eventually [went to] the Lister Hill Society asking for the money, and then fortuitously winded up presenting it at a time when Dr. Shamblin [a member of the board] was there, as well as others, who were intrigued with the idea, and we got generous donations," said Taylor in an interview.

The development of a state-of-the art computer laboratory became possible when the Shamblins came forward and offered to fund the lab in honor of their father, Dr. Roscoe Shamblin, who had been a pioneer member of the small physician group in Tuscaloosa in the 1930s. The new lab was built in a nicely furnished room on the fifth floor of the Education Tower at DCH and contained several high speed Dell computers, a scanner, video camera, a fax machine, and associated hardware and software.

"The computer," reflected Curry in a press release acknowledging the gift by the Shamblins in April of 2000, "is now an established tool in educating medical students, and it is increasingly important to the way we take care of patients. This gift of a state-of-the-art computer lab for our medical students here in Tuscaloosa is a guarantee that we can have them ready for this part of the twenty-first century medical practice. It is really a gift to the physicians and patients of the future."

The computer laboratory was an instant success and it was not long before the family practice residents requested a similar upgrade to their computer systems. Again the Shamblins offered to fund the new laboratory, also located in the Education Tower. The computer system, complete with six workstations, was opened in January 2001.

Dr. William Shamblin spoke about the value of the computer technology to the educational efforts at CCHS, noting that "it is utilized by both residents and students and we are delighted with that. This was a very positive cause that Dr. Michael Taylor first approached the Lister Hill board about. He asked for modest assistance in upgrading a system and eventually the Board decided to put in a state-of-the-art system."

Next, the college made improvements to the local computer network at the CMC, including the addition of newer and faster computers, a new server for the network, improved access to certain software applications, and training sessions for all personnel. This state-of-the-art information system was designed for everyone in the college, "from secretaries to faculty members, medical students, residents, and everybody in between," said Curry, noting the importance of everyone being in the network and "using technology in common." The subsequent purchase and installation of two new servers that support e-mail, file sharing, and an updated Web site for all four of its sites put the college in the "forefront of medical technology," according to Taylor.

The next step in modernizing the program was taken at the CMC, where efforts to modernize clinical care and teaching were made with the introduction of an electronic medical records system. The system, investigated and selected by McHattie, provided a "paperless" patient record that offered many advantages for rapid and accurate storage and retrieval of patient information, allowing the medical record to be immediately available to the patient care team. The system, with built-in mechanisms to protect confidentiality, provided instant access to laboratory results, medical histories, and treatment data. An additional benefit of the system was its ability to allow for the rapid analysis of many aspects of the entire group practice for management and clinical purposes. Implementation of the system began in winter 2002, and proceeded one department at a time so as to mitigate the impact on patient care. The system required that each physician learn to generate the patient record at the time of the visit, using a computer template and a notebook computer. The technology, predicted Curry, would "make it easier to do a better job for our patients and students."[86]

Technological strides were also made in the Health Sciences Library, where the staff had a long history of implementing various and innovative technologies in support of the mission of the college. One such advance was made in 1998 with the addition of a clinical digital library (CDL) that provided a monumental improvement in Internet usage for physicians, residents, and other health care workers. Developed by Dr. Steven McCall of the UA School of Library and Information Studies and his colleagues at the University of North Texas, the CDL yielded real-time access to reference materials to assist with patient care, providing a much-needed resource for the college. Although originally designed as a set of links to existing sites on the Internet, the system was enhanced over time to facilitate access to more than 1,000 clinical, patient, preventive medicine, and public health topics. The CDL also includes links to full-text journals to which the library subscribes, as well as electronic reference books (such as the *Physicians' Desk Reference,* an important but cumbersome book in its original hard-copy format). The CDL was designed simply and "aims at putting as few clicks as possible between the physician and the information he or she needs."[87]

Status of the Traditional Clinical Departments

One of the most visible signs of the progress made in the college since the early days was the improvement in undergraduate medical teaching at CCHS. Gone were the concerns by the LCME about the quality of medical education in Tuscaloosa. The teaching skills of the faculty at CCHS were now widely respected in the UA system, as evidenced by the many faculty members who were recognized by the UA National Alumni Association, which gives an annual award for excellence in teaching. Over the course of the history of the college, the award was given to five faculty members: Drs. Elizabeth Cockrum, Harry Knopke, James Leeper, Robert E. Pieroni, and William W. Winternitz. This represented a large percentage of a faculty that typically numbered only twenty-seven full-time members, but with a larger number of adjunct faculty members among the physicians in the community. A number of these physicians were outstanding teachers, identified as such by the medical students and residents who trained under them (Appendix B).

One area where the teaching has been strengthened over the years is in the Department of Internal Medicine, where both Pieroni and Winternitz hold their appointments. The CCHS program in internal medicine, under the leadership of Dean Curry as chair, was designed to teach students and residents to investigate and manage illness in adults. This process requires the ability to obtain a complete history; perform a complete and accurate physical examination; record obtained data properly in the format of the problem-oriented medical record; and communicate these data, both orally and in writing, to colleagues and others. To this end, the program's faculty, residents, and students engage in the systematic study of disease processes, the natural history of disease, the delivery of effective care, preventive medicine, and patient education. These educational efforts are supported by extensive clinical service in both inpatient and ambulatory settings.

The addition of a new faculty member in the 1990s added to the quality of the clinical teaching program; Dr. Cathy Gresham joined the college in 1991. A graduate of UASOM, she completed her clinical years at CCHS and then attended Carolina Medical Center in Charlotte, North Carolina, for her residency training before returning to Tuscaloosa. Appointed director of Medical Student Affairs in 1996, she supplemented the medical student program in a host of ways, interacting with students and working with colleagues in Birmingham to strengthen the clinical curriculum, which has recently become more elaborate. Teaching in Internal Medicine is also provided by Drs. Wheat and Vijaya Sundar. Likewise, a number of part-time faculty also strengthen the teaching, including Drs. Michael Robards, Lydia Stefanescu, and Albert White.

In late 1999 Dr. John Burnum retired from his private practice of thirty-five years and joined the college as its only Clinical Scholar in Residence. His clinical practice and his medical writings had brought him national visibility in the medical profession. His appointment, in the Department of Internal Medicine, was such that all third-year medical students, fourth-year medical students electively, and all residents would have some clinical experiences with him. His return to full-time academic pursuits at CCHS was a major boost to the teaching program in medicine.

The Department of Obstetrics/Gynecology witnessed many changes in the late 1990s and beyond. Leadership here has changed with the departures of Dr. Harvey Fair in 2000 and Dr. McHattie in 2001. But the basic goal of providing a top-quality educational experience to medical students remained the same. By 2002 teaching in the department was largely provided by Dr. Dwight Hooper, interim chair, assisted by Dr. Cindy Mathews, a graduate of the CCHS family practice residency and the obstetrics and gynecology fellowship. After joining the CCHS faculty in 2000, Hooper worked hard to strengthen this aspect of the undergraduate medical student curriculum, which includes training in obstetrics, office gynecologic procedures, and the common complications of fertility, pregnancy, and delivery. His goal, he explained in an interview, is to bring the department "more in line with what I think is the design and direction of the college as a whole, and that is being friendly to the primary care/family practice model of providing care."

One of Hooper's major efforts early in his tenure centered on recruiting others to the program. In late 2002 he was able to bring in Dr. Karl Hasik, a former member of the faculty who completed his residency at St. Louis University School of Medicine. In the meantime, he has used part-time faculty to assist with teaching, borrowing from the successful model established by the Department of Surgery.

A complementary objective of the CCHS program in the new millennium was to help reduce west Alabama's perinatal mortality rate by engaging in applied research and providing educational and backup services to the counties in the health service area of the college.

The Department of Surgery at CCHS continued to offer one of the most popular and successful teaching rotations under the leadership of Dr. Joseph Wallace, who trained at the Mayo Clinic. Wallace, a general surgeon, joined CCHS as chair of the department in 1995. He is assisted by Dr. Timothy W. Winkler, a former CCHS student who also took his residency at the Mayo Clinic and who teaches students and residents and assists in administrative matters.

In 2002 the surgical experience for CCHS students involved four weeks with a solo surgeon, which provides an excellent opportunity to have continuity with each patient, followed by four weeks in a larger group practice. All of the students also participate in an outpatient surgery setting. Fourth-year students may also choose to take an elective rotation with a surgical subspecialist such as urology, otolaryngology, orthopedics, or ophthalmology. Throughout the history of the program, the success of the teaching in this area has rested with the many local surgeons who donated their time to the teaching program, as well as many part-time faculty members.

The Department of Pediatrics, chaired by Dr. Michael Taylor, has also continuously provided a strong tradition of teaching. Longtime faculty members Drs. David Hefelfinger and Elizabeth Cockrum were joined by Dr. Ashley Evans, who joined the full-time faculty in 1994, and by Dr. Karen Burgess in 2001 after completing her degree at CCHS and her residency training in the pediatrics department at UASOM.

Throughout the history of the college, this department has demonstrated its total commitment to teaching pediatrics to students and residents. Hefelfinger, as the initial chair, successfully recruited like-minded professionals over the years and the tradition of outstanding teaching has continued, but with new skills added in medical information and clinical research.

Furthermore, the pediatrics department has maintained a close alliance with the parent department in Birmingham over the past thirty years. Specialty clinics in cardiology and sickle-cell disease take place on a monthly basis, staffed by specialists from UASOM. An allergy clinic staffed by pediatric allergists Drs. John F. Dishuck and Steven G. Helms, adjunct associate professors, provided CCHS students with important exposure to the issues associated with childhood allergies and their treatment.

In 2002 medical students at CCHS were taught psychiatry by a group of four faculty members under the leadership of Dr. Elizabeth Rand, department chair, who joined CCHS in 1986. The main thrust of the teaching program has been to give students a solid experience in general adult psychiatry in both hospital and office settings. Furthermore, students receive training in geriatric psychiatry at the V.A. Hospital in Tuscaloosa and in child psychiatry at the Maude Whatley Clinic.

The psychiatry and neurology rotations are concurrent, but with separate facilities. The eight-week rotation in psychiatry continues to include three weeks of neurology. Teaching in this area has been strengthened in recent years with the addition of neurologist Eugene Marsh, who joined the CCHS faculty full-time in 2001 as associate dean of Academic Affairs, after having been on the faculty part-time for eight years. While in private practice in Tuscaloosa he acted as a preceptor to both residents and medical students from CCHS. The offer from CCHS allowed him an opportunity "to teach more and be on the ground floor for developing curriculum," he said. He has been recognized by the CCHS students numerous times for his teaching ability. In 2002 he directed the clerkship in neurology with Drs. Ben H. Lucy, III, Arturo J. Otero, James D. Geyer, Daniel C. Potts, Thomas K. Emig, Brian K. Hogan, and Fernando Franco serving as adjunct faculty members.

One of the most exciting aspects of the psychiatry program at CCHS, reflected Rand in an interview, was the opportunity to have an impact on primary care physicians. "As a psychiatrist, I can only affect a few people, but these primary care physicians are seeing the majority of the people who have mental illness," she said. Therefore, one of her goals as chair has been to shift the student and resident curricula toward outpatient work and "to try to address the recognition of mental disorders along with, obviously, how to treat them once you have a case." In this regard, Rand and her colleagues have worked with both residents and students.

In 2002 the Department of Psychiatry and Behavioral Medicine was staffed by Rand and three full-time faculty members, Drs. Nancy Rubin, L. Roger Lacy, and Melissa C. Kuhajda. Rubin joined the faculty in 1990 as the first clinical psychologist in the department and helped to foster a strong relationship with the UA Department of Psychology while developing a large service in direct patient care at the CMC and teaching family practice residents. Lacy was a CCHS student before completing an internship at UASOM in internal medicine and completing his residency in psychiatry at the Menninger Clinic in Topeka, Kansas. He joined the department in 1994 and has assisted with a major change in the curriculum that moved from an emphasis on institutionalized patients to community-based patients in hospital and outpatient settings. Kuhajda, with a Ph.D. in clinical psychology from UASOM, joined the faculty in 2000. Five adjunct faculty members supplement the teaching program, including Drs. Carlos Berry, Sylvia Colon, Sanjay Singh, Gary Newsom, and Kamal Raisani. Rand has been successful in providing both students and residents with a well-rounded learning experience by using part-time faculty and facilities outside the college. The department has also produced research pertinent to primary medical care.

A unique aspect of the CCHS program has always been the attention paid to community medicine, and the college leadership has consistently emphasized this important component of medical education. Although the curriculum changed over the years and the length of the community medicine rotation varied, CCHS students have long had excellent exposure to the concepts of community medicine as envisioned by Dean Willard at the inception of the program. In 2000 the Department of Community and Behavioral Medicine was renamed the Department of Community and Rural Medicine to reflect more accurately the emphasis on the rural service and education component of the college. In the new millennium, the department consists of Dr. Leeper, Dr. Wheat, and the newest member, Dr. John Higginbotham. A native of Alabama, Higginbotham received an M.P.H. from the UAB School of Public Health in 1986 and a Ph.D. in preventive medicine and behavioral epidemiology from the University of Texas Medical Branch at Galveston in 1992. He joined the department in 1999 as an associate professor; he also holds an adjunct faculty position at the UAB School of Public Health. Leadership in the department was long provided by Leeper, who served as chair of the department from 1987 until 2001 when he stepped down as chair and Higginbotham was asked to serve as interim chair.

With the new emphasis on rural medicine that came with Dean Curry's arrival, the community medicine experience has been retooled to allow the students more latitude in their assignments. Third-year students are required to conduct a research project in a rural community that examines the larger issues of health in these areas and the kind of intervention that the community might put in place to address these issues. This rotation is done on the heels of their family medicine clerkship, which is done in the office of a rural preceptor in the same community. In this way, the students get to know and explore a rural community, spending time with community leaders and health care personnel. The rotation has become more rewarding, stated Leeper in an interview, who reported getting "glowing reports from the students about the experience." He noted that the community medicine rotation was one of the few in the entire medical school curriculum that allowed the students to be out in the community, to manage their own time, and to explore a topic on their own.

"It's very different from anything else," he said, "a lot of them see it as a very welcome experience, a break in their routine of what they've been doing—out of the clinic, out of the hospital that they've spent all their time in—and they have a very different angle."

Another advantage of the experience, Leeper went on to note, was that it opened the eyes of students who may not have witnessed what life can be like in poor, underserved areas. "I think a lot of medical students have led fairly privileged lives and have never seen this side of life and what poverty does to people and how people make decisions about medication versus food and that sort of thing. And so they come back with a real dose of reality and find that extremely valuable. It's going to carry over into everything else they do in medicine."

It is this rotation that helped distinguish CCHS from many other medical school programs. In fact, students from other universities throughout the country have come to Alabama to participate in this unique community medicine program. "The Department of Community and Rural Medicine's rural medicine rotation has improved over the past three years," noted Higginbotham in 2002. "It's become a lot more specific in its requirement and its expectation, and I think it's provided increased benefits for the students."

The CCHS student population has continued to grow and change over the thirty-year history of the college. Students from UASOM respond to the reputation that CCHS had built and they regularly sign on to the Tuscaloosa program with enthusiasm. Dean Deal noted that the strength of the program lies in attracting faculty who had a "genuine interest in medical students and medical student teaching." He also noted that the structure of the program at CCHS allows much closer contact between students and faculty, which is unusual in larger schools with a large array of subspecialists as full-time faculty.

Dean Curry noted that it is the quality of the teaching that makes the CCHS program stand out. "I think it shows in the way students look at this place," he noted in an interview. "They select it because of that, even though it may be an inconvenience to their family situation to relocate from Birmingham. I think it's a testimony to the dedication of the faculty to good teaching here, that's really the heritage of CCHS." To that end, Dr. Cathy Gresham, director of Medical Student Affairs at CCHS, noted there is no longer concern about the number of students who elect to come to CCHS, as the number is sufficient to fill the available teaching resources. This differs considerably from the early years when CCHS faculty were concerned that there would be too few students to fill the teaching service.

But the excellence of the medical student program at CCHS has not been taken for granted and in 2002, under the leadership of Marsh in his role as associate dean of Academic Affairs, the teaching programs in each department have been further strengthened. Members of a newly organized education committee conducted a systematic review of every clerkship, experience, and program to assess its value to the students who came to CCHS. "As good as we are," explained Curry, "we need to be sure we're staying current, not only with technology and teaching techniques, but with the needs of our students and with the changes in content in the specialties."

A key initiative in this regard has been a focus on faculty development and Marsh's role here proved to be critical. One of his goals has been to help the CCHS faculty build on their experience to become even better instructors and to expand the number participating in clinical research.

Family Medicine and the State of the Residency

The quality of instruction in the college's family practice residency program has been extremely important in the building of the CCHS reputation, and in this regard the faculty of the college was strong. As a result, this keystone of CCHS has been fulfilling the need for more family doctors in Alabama (see map on page 100). By 1999, the twenty-fifth year of the program, there were 258 graduates, making it one of the most productive programs in the Southeast. By this time leadership for the residency was again provided by Dr. Samuel E. Gaskins, who agreed to serve as director of the program again after Dr. Marc Armstrong resigned the position to focus on his duties as associate dean for Clinical Affairs. Over a period of more than twenty years as residency director, Gaskins had seen a great deal of change as the program evolved with the times; he served the program well.

In 1999 another key position in the college was filled as Dr. Alan Blum agreed to join the Department of Family Medicine as the Gerald Leon Wallace Endowed Chair in Family Medicine for CCHS, one of only twenty family medicine endowed chairs in the country. Blum, a nationally recognized expert in the health hazards of tobacco use, had a broad experience in academic family medicine. With a medical degree from Emory University School of Medicine, Blum completed an internship at McGill University School of Medicine in Montreal, Quebec, and a residency at the University of Miami School of Medicine in Florida, the first accredited family medicine program in the country. It was in Florida that he first became interested in the ravages of tobacco use on the public's health and he began speaking and writing on the topic. He later founded an organization called Doctors Ought to Care (DOC) to stimulate physicians to become more vocal about the risks associated with smoking. He also founded—and continues to direct—the Center for the Study of Tobacco and Society, the world's largest archive of material documenting the history of tobacco use and the influence of tobacco advertising on society, which is now based at CCHS. Blum was recruited from the family practice program of the Baylor College of Medicine in Houston, Texas, where he taught for twelve years.

The new millennium brought additional personnel changes for the program. In 2001, a longtime faculty member, Dr. Bobbi Adcock, retired after a prolonged illness. Her role as director of the student program in family medicine had been crucial; she initiated and supervised an out-patient clinic where medical students could obtain longitudinal experience with their own patients for an entire year. She was recognized by students and residents as an exceptional clinical teacher. Not long after her departure two new faculty members were added to the department, Dr. Laura Satcher and Dr. Chelley Alexander. Satcher, a graduate of the CCHS residency and the Obstetrics/Gynecology fellowship with a medical degree from the University of South Alabama, eagerly embarked on several research projects and agreed to coordinate medical student affairs for the department. Alexander also graduated from the residency and assumed the position of the assistant residency director after Robert Ireland stepped down from this position.

In 2001 a change in leadership also occurred in the Department of Family Medicine when Dr. Jerry McKnight stepped down from his position as chair, a post he had held for six years. In his place Dr. William Owings agreed to serve as interim chair. Owings had a long association with the college serving as the preceptor to dozens of students and residents since the inception of the program in Tuscaloosa.

As the personnel in the department changed, so did other aspects of the program. In the late 1990s a change occurred in the selection of residents at CCHS due to a nationwide decrease in interest in family medicine. Consequently, the percentage of U.S. medical students filling the family practice residencies was falling consistently and attrition of the residency programs was occurring throughout the country. Administrators struggled to fill the residency class each year. Some classes did not fill, such as the class that was recruited for 1999, making the schedule more demanding for those who did join the program. In light of the difficulties experienced by this class, the college administration considered downsizing the program from its traditional configuration of thirty-six residents, that is, twelve per class. Many factors had to be weighed: the presence of only one residency at the hospital and its importance to that organization, the size of the hospital, the number of medical students in the program and the integrated and structured success of the team on-call system. In the end, in a nod to the long-standing and excellent track record of the program, the administration opted to retain the size of the program, but with revisions, including an expansion of the recruiting pool to include graduates of osteopathic U.S. medical schools and international medical graduates. This decision caused a slightly higher attrition rate in the program, but a number of international medicine graduates proved to be solid in their performance and several came to be leaders in the program.

New Life for Community Medicine

In spite of the ongoing challenges associated with financial constraints and the recruiting of residents, many aspects of the program continued to grow and prosper.

In 2000 the department organized and hosted the first annual Alabama Rural Health Conference in concert with the university's health-related colleges, including the College of Human Environmental Sciences, Capstone College of Nursing, the College of Commerce and Business Administration, and the School of Social Work. According to Curry, who conceptualized the conference, the meeting provided a vehicle for these organizations to explore ways to "make life better" for those living in rural Alabama. Thus the two-day meeting provided a forum in which pertinent rural health issues—ranging from access to clean water to transportation issues to HIV prevention—could be discussed.[88] The intent of the two-day meeting, according to organizer Dr. John Higginbotham, was to foster relationships between individuals and institutions, identify obstacles to progress and promote the development of creative, collaborative long-term strategies. More than two hundred people from rural communities, churches, health agencies, and educational organizations attended. Organizations such as Blue Cross/Blue Shield of Alabama provided financial support. A number of statewide organizations associated with health issues provided generous support for this conference, which was to be held annually from this point on. "This annual conference has proved to be a major step toward fulfilling one of the dreams of President Mathews and Dean Willard in 1972."

Shortly after his arrival at CCHS, Higginbotham was named director of the Institute for Rural Health Research (IRHR), a CCHS organization that developed from the Research Consulting Lab that was formed in the 1980s by Leeper. In 2001 the program evolved further and was renamed the Institute for Rural Health Research. Although housed in CCHS, the program is a collaborative effort that encompasses the College of Arts and Sciences, Human Environmental Sciences, the Capstone College of Nursing, the School of Social Work, and the College of Commerce and Business Administration. Through the institute CCHS is able to reach out to CCHS faculty as well as faculty in other colleges and assist them with obtaining funds for research.

In 2001 another program was added to help further expand the efforts to build a medical pipeline in Alabama. In an effort to reach out to minority groups who had long been underrepresented in medicine (and the sciences in general), Wheat and his colleagues established the Minority Rural Health Pipeline. Funded by the Robert Wood Johnson Southern Rural Access Program in Alabama and the Alabama Family Practice Rural Health Board, the program offers support, both financial and academic, to minority students who demonstrate interest and the capability to seek a career in medicine.

Moving Forward on the New Building

Of all the developments that occurred at CCHS during its first twenty-five years, few generated the kind of excitement that accompanied the planning for the new building. In September of 2001, the university's board of trustees approved a bond issue for the new facility with the understanding that the Capstone Health Services Foundation would repay the bond money over a period of time if private donors did not respond sufficiently. But the bond issue itself was not sufficient to pay the total cost of the $12.9 million building and concerns about how to obtain the necessary funding abounded.

In 2001 a special fund was organized to honor Mrs. Betty Shirley, a local resident and longtime proponent of improved mental health services in the community. She had consistently supported the work of the psychiatry clinic at the university, and the money raised in her name provided the funds needed to build the new mental health clinic to be located in the new CMC. It was named for her.

Additional funding for the new building also came from the sale of the educational tower at DCH, which the hospital agreed to purchase when the teaching functions there could be accommodated in the new building. This integral part of the physical structure of the hospital will be used by DCH for a variety of purposes.

An unexpected new source of support came from the Medicare Trust Fund, which will provide additional funds for the residency program. These funds provide support for medical education, but they do not add to the cost of Medicare services for patients.

As funding issues were being resolved, the physical shape, size, and location of the building were being formulated. CCHS administrators worked with the architects to design a building that would provide an optimal environment for patient care, research, and service. The 77,000-square-foot building was to be placed at the corner of Fifth Avenue East and University Boulevard on land owned by the university. This location, while still in close proximity to the hospital, provided much better visibility for the college, which had long suffered from a lack of recognition in the Tuscaloosa community. "Sometimes people forget we have medical education here in Tuscaloosa and that we're part of the School of Medicine," said Curry.[89]

A groundbreaking for the building was held in November 2002. In attendance were U.S. Senator Richard Shelby, UASOM dean Dr. William Deal, UA interim president Dr. Barry Mason, Dr. Malcolm Portera, chancellor of the university system, Dr. Nancy Barrett, provost of the university, Judge John England of the UA board of trustees, Dr. David Rice, vice president for medical affairs at DCH, deans emeriti Dr. Wilmer Coggins and Dr. Roland Ficken and a host of supporters of the college.

At the ceremony held on that November afternoon, Curry noted that the building would bring most of the CCHS faculty and staff together in one facility for the first time in thirty years.

Furthermore, he noted, that "as this building rises, so does the visibility of the College of Community Health Sciences and the School of Medicine Tuscaloosa."

The promise of a new building brought hope for a solid future and a strengthened commitment to providing primary care physicians for underserved areas and underserved people.

Epilogue

The thirtieth year of CCHS brought changes for the faculty, staff, and its supporters. The dawning of a new decade brought the hope—finally—that the college was on stable ground, that it was on the right track, that its future was secure, and that it was making critical strides in its mission of providing primary care doctors for Alabama. "We have moved from survival," noted Dean Curry, "to significance."[90]

The people in the program have built valuable relationships across the campus and across the state, from county health departments to other colleges on the UA campus. The bond between the college and DCH, for example, is stronger than ever, thanks to a mutual respect and understanding. Support from the hospital administration and its medical staff is greater than ever in both tangible and intangible ways. The combined efforts of both institutions are evident throughout the region, most notably in the graduates of the residency program who are now practicing in the state. Willard's fervent desire that the hospital staff would one day "come around" and recognize the value of this educational endeavor has truly come to pass.

By the year 2002, under Curry's leadership, the seeds sown by Willard, Mathews, and so many others in the state had not only germinated, they were in full bloom. The results of this effort are impressive and a source of pride for many. Nearly 500 students have completed their medical education at CCHS. Of these, 48 percent chose careers in primary care, including pediatrics, family practice, and internal medicine. The results of UASOM's two branch campus programs, Tuscaloosa and Huntsville, in encouraging students to choose family practice as their career endeavor is especially encouraging in the light of national trends over the past twenty-five years. In Tuscaloosa, 20 percent of the graduates have chosen family practice; in Huntsville, 23 percent; even in Birmingham, 8 percent of those students who elected to complete their four years on the main campus chose family practice. This is in stark contrast to the well-known research institutions, such as Emory, Duke, and Johns Hopkins. There, fewer than one percent of the graduates chose family practice.

But CCHS has not been alone. Over the past thirty years, a number of medical schools in the Southeast have also demonstrated a concern for addressing the shortage of doctors in nonurban areas. Data through the year 2000 show that some of them have been successful in numbers comparable to CCHS and UASOM Huntsville. Among those that encouraged family practice as a specialty choice, we see the following outcomes: the University of Kentucky, 15 percent; the University of Mississippi, 16 percent; the University of South Alabama, 16 percent; Mercer, 27 percent.

It is apparent that medical schools which are part of academic centers where biomedical research and high-technology medicine are principal goals do not encourage medical students to choose family practice or general internal medicine as careers. The experience in Alabama proves that small clinical branch campuses, such as Huntsville and Tuscaloosa, can succeed in accomplishing this divergent but invaluable goal. From the beginning of these two programs in 1975, through 2002, the total residency program output has been 290 in Tuscaloosa and 265 in Huntsville.

Over the past thirty years the complexities of first-rate health care delivery have created challenges that require technologies even at the interface between the doctor and the patient—between the providers and the users. These technologies can best be developed and analyzed in community-based programs such as CCHS, where the patient population reflects a community, and where continuity of care is provided. Implementation of an electronic medical record, as is now underway at CCHS, is one example of an effort to solve the increasing complexity of health care delivery by a more efficient record system that lends itself to a continued analysis of outcomes.

The college's family practice residency shows similarly excellent outputs. By 2002 the college had trained 290 family doctors. Many of these, almost 52 percent, have gone on to practice in Alabama; today one in eight family physicians in the state completed his or her training at CCHS (see map on page 100). Many other graduates have settled in neighboring southeastern states. Such results are particularly impressive in light of the declining number of students who chose family practice residencies.[91] The program is working. The availability of medical care in Alabama's underserved counties has improved, and those who have been part of the mission can be proud of what has been done.

An unexpected benefit to the college has come about in the past two decades. Early concerns about the parochialism of the program, educating Alabama medical students to practice in Alabama and training medical graduates to practice family medicine in Alabama, might deprive both students and faculty of broader experiences in medical education and medical practice. Several factors operated to quell these concerns. Many of the medical students chose to complete their specialty training in other academic medical centers. Some of them chose to return to CCHS in later years as faculty members. In a small faculty such as this, even one faculty member who brings experiences and insights from other institutions can make a difference.

Graduates of the residency program have become leaders in organized medicine and in academic medicine in gratifying numbers (see Appendix E). Many of the former residents have become mainstays as preceptors in both family and community medicine, and in the Supervised Practice Experience for the residents (Appendices C and D).

The college continues to look ahead at how things can be made even better, for even today a shortage of primary care doctors exists in the state. The state's department of public health estimates that the state is still short about two hundred such doctors. The establishment and nourishment of the medical pipeline in Alabama is a start. By focusing on promising rural high school students, the program offers hope that even more medical students will soon become part of the solution to the rural physician manpower shortage. The past successes are encouraging: 274 high-school students from fifty-nine Alabama counties have now completed the Rural Health Scholars program. The five-year Rural Medical Scholars program was beginning to see similarly positive results after its fifth year of operation; by 2002 seventeen medical graduates had completed the program. Of these, twelve selected residencies in primary care and ten of the seventeen committed to rural service scholarships, for which they receive generous scholarship support in return for a commitment to practice in rural Alabama.

A focused effort to expand the research and scholarly activities of the faculty continues. In recent years those efforts have more than doubled, as measured by grant money and research publications. By 2002 the total amount of grant and contract support received by the relatively small CCHS faculty was $26,887,450. Over the course of the history of the college such funds have offered much more than just external fiscal support; the resulting research offers concrete results for the people of Alabama in large and small ways. Clinical studies now underway include studies of infant mortality, treatment of asthma in children, treatment of post-traumatic stress disorder, barriers to prostate cancer screening, and several others. These studies can help provide practical solutions to health care issues facing the citizens of the state, while providing faculty, students, and residents opportunities to grow professionally and acquire valuable research skills that may well be useful in their careers.

The rural health mission of the college continues to be broadened. Ties with rural communities are being strengthened through such activities as the annual rural health conferences, which establishes and encourages ongoing ties among health-related agencies at the state, regional, and local level. Increasingly, CCHS is becoming recognized for the innovations of its faculty in this regard, and this is expected to continue.

In *Mini-Med: The Role of Regional Campuses in U.S. Medical Education,* the authors summarize the difference between main and regional campuses.[92]

> A dean at one of the regional campuses questioned whether his
> program was an island or a peninsula. The conclusion was that
> it was an isthmus, or better, a bridge—a bridge "at the nexus of
> education and patient care, of academician and clinician, of ivory
> tower and community. . . . [Regional campuses] are to be valued
> for expanding opportunities, experiences, and missions, and for
> bridging the oftentimes wide gulf between town and gown."

As one studies the history of the college, through its many ups and downs, one thing becomes clear: the goal set in the 1960s by the Alabama legislature to place more doctors in Alabama's towns and rural areas is being achieved. Through the dedication and determination of a small group of administrators, doctors, legislators, alumni, and other supporters throughout the state and region, CCHS is producing primary care doctors for the state. And this benefits us all.

Appendix A:
Number of Graduates* of the
Residency Program, by Year,
with Chief Residents

Graduating Year	Number of Graduates	Chief Residents
1976	2	Michael McBrearty
1977	4	Nicolas A. Knight
1978	12	J. Rickey Gober
1979	11	Herbert A. Stone
1980	11	Rodney V. Snead
1981	8	Thomas J. Burchett
		W. Larry Tucker
1982	13	S. Catherine Huggins
		J. Glenn Peters
1983	8	David L. Barnes
		Marc F. Fisher
1984	12	W. Reid Bell
		E. Edward Martin
1985	11	J. Trent Beaton
		Randall R. Hankins
1986	12	Steve R. Lovelady
		Norman G. Stevens
1987	13	S. Randall Easterling
		Jimmy S. Tu

*Although the residency is not a degree granting program it provides the terminal formal educational experience for residents who satisfactorily complete the three years. They are then qualified for the national specialty board examination in family medicine.

1988	12	Billy M. Pickering
		Thomas J. Smitherman
1989	12	Vance G. Blackburn
		James W. Ervin
1990	13	Ray H. Brown
		Brian W. Elrod
1991	13	John B. Crider
		Charles M. Eddins
1992	12	Lisa D. Columbia
		Edgar N. Donahoe
1993	9	M. Blane Schilling
		R. Kelvin Sherman
1994	9	Craig M. Buettner
		Christopher M. McGee
1995	13	Jeffrey M. Donohue
		F. Wayne Kelly
1996	14	Dan Moore
		Angela Powell
1997	10	Martin Harvey
		Stuart Hendon
1998	10	Kent Kanatani
		Chris Sward
1999	14	Lucius (Beau) Freeman
		Amy Shenkenberg
2000	12	Michael Elliott
		Jeff Laubenthal
2001	12	Brad Gaspard
		Natasha Harder
2002	8	Jennifer Burdette
		Shane Phillips

Total Graduates: 290

Appendix B:
Teaching Awards Presented by Students to CCHS Faculty and Residents, 1977–2003

At the Honors Banquet signaling the end of the academic year for the senior students, they give an award to the most outstanding teacher that year. The third-year students do the same. The two classes are exposed to a different array of instructors over the two years. It is unusual for one physician to be chosen as the outstanding one by both classes in the same year.

Teaching Awards to Faculty

The following faculty members have been so honored since 1978. A few have been honored in more than one year. Exactly half of these recipients have been part-time or volunteer faculty.

Department of Surgery
R. Joe Burlson
Gabriel Fernandez
H. Gorden King (3)
John Shamblin
William Shamblin
Arthur F. Snyder
Lee Thomas
Joseph C. Wallace

Department of Medicine
Sahria Kamal
Dennis Delgado
John Burnum (2)
Michael Lindberg
Patrick McCue* (5)
Robert Pieroni
Mark Ricketts (2)
Michael Robards
William W. Winternitz (3)

*Dr. Patrick McCue was medical director of the Tuscaloosa Veterans Affairs Medical Center. After he had won the award five times, it was named for him and he became ineligible to further receive it.

Department of Pediatrics
Elizabeth Cockrum (2)
Ashley Evans
Thomas Farmer
Michael Taylor

Anesthesiology
Joseph Hill
Eugene Mangieri

Neurology
E. Eugene Marsh (7)

Obstetrics and Gynecology
Mary Joyce McGinnis

Radiation Oncology
Shelby Sanford

Teaching Awards to Residents

Each year the medical students recognize the family practice resident who they view as the best teacher.

1977—John B. Sullivan
1978—John B. Sullivan
1979—Herbert A. Stone
1980—Richard E. Matis

1981—Martha H. Crenshaw
1982—William Philip Smith
1983—John V. Murray
1984—Robert E. Lahasky
1985—Joe A. Dunn
1986—Steve R. Lovelady
1987—
1988—Billy M. Pickering
1989—Spencer J. Coleman

1990—John B. Crider
1991—Edgar N. Donahoe
1992—Edgar N. Donahoe
1993—Christoopher E. McGee
1994—Jeffrey A. Donohue
1995—Angela A. Powell
1996—Angela A. Powell
1997—Kent Kanatani
1998—Lisa Sward
1999—Melvin A. Williams
2000—Brad J. Gaspard
2001—Brad J. Gaspard
2002—Salih O. Faldon

Appendix C:
Rural Physician Preceptors for Family Medicine and Community Medicine

Volunteer physicians have made major contributions to the mandatory rural health and community medicine rotations throughout the life of the college. More than one hundred physicians practicing in small towns have served as preceptors for CCHS students. Certain physicians have proved to be more accepting of medical students in their practice, and sometimes in their home, for one month or longer. These have been very popular choices for the students.

From 1975 to 1980 five physicians accepted almost two-thirds of the students into their practice.* They were Dr. Rucker Staggers in Eutaw, Greene County; Dr. William Owings in Centreville, Bibb County; Dr. Richard Rutland and Dr. Jon Sanford in Fayette, Fayette County; and Dr. Robert Holcomb in Hamilton, Marion County.

In the next decade, from 1981–1990, graduates of the CCHS residency program practicing in nearby small towns welcomed medical students into their individual practices. Student numbers in the Tuscaloosa program increased substantially during this decade. Former residents John Brandon in Gordo, Pickens County; Sandral Hullett in Eutaw, Greene County; Gary Magouirk in Fayette, Fayette County; and Larry Skelton in Moundville, Hale County, served as preceptors for a large number of students and residents. Dr. McBrearty** also accepted more than his share of students although his practice in Fairhope, Baldwin County, was more than two hundred miles from Tuscaloosa.

Dr. William Curry, practicing in Carrollton, Pickens County, also accepted a number of students and residents in his practice. He was well

*There were forty-four students in five years.
**The first person to complete the residency program at CCHS

known to them because he was periodically serving as an attending on the CCHS service at DCH Regional Medical Center.

Other preceptors who accepted four or more students during this decade were Dr. James N. Hall, Jr., in Trussville, Jefferson County; Dr. Samuel Roberts and Dr. Carol Johnson (a CCHS graduate) in Alabaster, Shelby County; Dr. George G. Thomas in Greensboro, Hale County; Dr. Blane Schilling and Dr. David Tuten in Carrollton, Pickens County.

A number of students chose to take their preceptorships in foreign countries; this was in part due to the interest of Dr. Robert Northrup, chairman of the Department of Community Medicine, and his contacts in international medicine, but also through contacts made by other faculty physicians. Students studied in India, Indonesia, Bangladesh, Europe, Africa, the Caribbean Islands, and South America. One senior student, Larry Mayes, died from encephalitis soon after reporting for duty in Zimbabwe at a church mission, but this tragic event did not cause others to avoid experience in third-world medicine. Mayes was awarded the M.D. degree posthumously. His fellow students established an annual award in his name to go to an outstanding student.

Over the next decade, a committed cadre of preceptors continued to serve the larger number of students, but some volunteers resigned or moved to other locations. Graduates of the residency program continued to be the major choices for both students and residents.

The following preceptors continue to accept medical students for their family medicine and community medicine rotations (current through 2002).

Current Preceptors, with location by city and county

Regina M. Benjamin	Steve Paul Furr	John Smith
Bayou La Batre, Mobile	Jackson, Clarke	Oneonta, Blount
John Boggess	Samuel Gillespie	Judson Smith
Scottsboro, Jackson	Moulton, Lawrence	Jasper, Walker
Charles Bradford	Katherine Hensleigh	Kenneth Strother
Scottsboro, Jackson	Butler, Greenville	Opelika, Lee

Tonya Bradley
Tallassee, Elmore

Carol Johnson
Alabaster, Shelby

James Temple
Alexander City,
Tallaoosa

John Brandon
Gordo, Pickens

John Meigs
Centreville, Bibb

James Tuck
Pell City, St. Clair

Clay Davis
Phoenix City, Russell

Lata Patil
Centreville, Bibb

Maria Villarreal
Brewton, Escambia

Garry A. Dillard
Phoenix City, Russell

Harry Phillips
Columbiana, Shelby

Walter Wilson
Pinson, Jefferson

Angelia Elliot
Cullman, Cullman

Jerry Robinson
Boaz, Marshall

Steven Winston
Fairhope, Baldwin

Beau Freeman
Prattville, Autauga

Larry Skelton
Moundville, Hale

Appendix D:
Physician Preceptors for Residents' Supervised Practice Experience

The Supervised Practice Experience (SPE) for family practice residents has been a required part of this program since its inception in 1974. Many graduates of the residency program have entered practice in surrounding rural areas and in Tuscaloosa, and many of them have served as preceptors for the SPE, for residents coming along behind them. While not all of these practices are rural, they offer other aspects of primary care such as more diverse patient populations.

One of the strengths of community-based programs in medical education is the use of private practitioners for teaching medical students and residents. Family practice residency programs usually try to maintain an on-site office facility that mimics a private doctor's office for a solo or small group practice. Over time, however, these on-site practices become institutionalized in a variety of ways, becoming less like nonacademic settings. For this reason practice experiences in other settings become even more valuable.

The following list includes the volunteer family physicians, many of whom also accept medical students for their required rural family practice and community medicine experience.

All of the physicians listed below are regularly selected for the SPE. Those who are not graduates of this residency are identified by an asterisk.

We recognize several of these volunteer physicians who have students or residents in their practice more often than not: John Brandon, Gary Magouirk, William Owings, and Larry Skelton. They have served the college in this capacity and many others over the years. Dr. Rucker Staggers, in Eutaw, Alabama, gave generously of his time and effort in the early years of the college, as did Dr. Richard Rutland in Fayette, and Dr. Sandral Hullett in Eutaw. Dr. William Owings was preceptor to at least thirty students or residents in his thirty years of practice in Centreville. He now serves as interim chair of the Department of Family Medicine, having retired from his practice.

John Brandon	Garry Magouirk	Richard Rutland*
Craig Buettner	Cindy Mathews	Blane Schilling
Jennifer Burdette	William McClanahan*	Vernon Scott
Audra Busenlehner	John Meigs*	Larry Skelton
John Dishuck*	William O. Owings*	Rucker Staggers*
Joseph Fritz	Norbet T. Perrett	David Tuten
Kevin Katona	Harry Phillips*	Raymond Ufford*
Jeff Laubenthal	Jimmy Robinson	

Appendix E:
Graduates of Residency Program Who Have Become Leaders in Organized Medicine and/or Academic Medicine

Former residents who have served as:

President of the Alabama Academy of Family Physicians
Michael McBrearty
John E. Brandon
Gary W. Magouirk
F. Keith Bufford
M. Blane Schilling

President of the Georgia Academy of Family Physicians
S. Catherine Huggins

President of the Louisiana Academy of Family Physicians
Robert E. Lahasky
E. Edward Martin

Academic Positions
Richard Streiffer, Chair, Family and Community Medicine, Tulane University, New Orleans, LA
E. Edward Martin, Chair, Family Medicine, Oschner Clinic Foundation, New Orleans, LA
Jerry McKnight, Chair, Family Medicine, CCHS
Robert B. Ireland, Associate Professor, Family Medicine, CCHS
Chelley Alexander, Assistant Professor, Family Medicine, CCHS
Laura Satcher, Assistant Professor, Family Medicine, CCHS
Melissa Behringer, Assistant Professor, Family Medicine, UASOM, Huntsville

Marcia Chesebro, Associate Professor, Family Medicine, UASOM, Huntsville

John B. Sullivan, Jr., Associate Dean for Clinical Affairs, University of Arizona, School of Medicine

Notes

1. Ad Hoc Committee on Education for Family Practice. "Meeting the Challenge of Family Practice" [known as "the Willard report"] (Chicago: Council of Medical Education, American Medical Association, 1966), p. 7.

2. G. Gayle Stephens, *The Intellectual Basis of Family Practice* (Tucson, AZ: Winter Publishing Co., 1982), p. 8.

3. Kenneth Ludmerer, *Time to Heal* (Oxford: Oxford University Press, 1999), p. 4.

4. William Warren Rogers, Robert David Ward, Leah Rawls Atkins, and Wayne Flynt, *Alabama: History of a Deep South State* (Tuscaloosa: The University of Alabama Press, 1994), p. 365.

5. Kenneth Ludmerer, *Learning to Heal* (New York: Basic Books, Inc., 1985), p. 18.

6. Reginald Horsman, *Josiah Nott of Mobile* (Baton Rouge: Louisiana State University, 1987), p. 11.

7. Howard Holley, *A History of Medicine in Alabama* (University: The University of Alabama Press, 1982), p. 65. This is the equivalent of $102,000 in year 2000 dollars.

8. Ibid., p. 99.

9. Ibid., p. 241.

10. Ludmerer, *Time to Heal*, p. 5.

11. Holley, p. 91.

12. Abraham Flexner, *Medical Education in the United States and Canada* (New York: The Carnegie Foundation, 1910), p. viii.

13. Mark D. Hiatt, "Around the continent in 180 days: The controversial journey of Abraham Flexner," *The Pharos*, Winter 1999, pp. 18–24.

14. Flexner, p. ix.

15. Holley, p. 94.

16. Suzanne Rau Wolfe, *The University of Alabama: A Pictorial History* (University: University of Alabama Press, 1983), p. 128.

17. Stuart Graves, speech delivered to annual banquet of Medical Association of the State of Alabama, April 22, 1936, Montgomery, Alabama.

18. A. W. Blair, "Spider poisoning: Experimental study of the effects of the bite of the female *Latrodectus mactans* in man," *Archives of Internal Medicine*, Vol. 54, no. 6, December 1934, pp. 831–43.

19. Ledmerer, *Time to Heal*, p. 126.

20. Author unknown, "University medical school dates back to 1859," *Crimson White*, 1931, p. 33.

21. *Crimson White*, p. 34.

22. Holley, p. 106.

23. Speagle, Scott M. "By process of elimination: The political decisions behind locating a four-year medical school in Birmingham," *The Vulcan Historical Review*, Vol. 2, Spring 1998, p. 58.

24. Ludmerer, *Time to Heal*, p.xxii.

25. Ibid., p. 196.

26. The Graduate Education of Physicians: The Report of the Citizens Commission on Graduate Medical Education. (Chicago: American Medical Association, 1966), p. 35.

27. Willard report, p. 7.

28. Ibid., p. 15.

29. Kurt W. Deuschle and Frederick Eberson, "Community medicine comes of age," *J. Med. Educ*, Vol. 43, December 1968, p. 1229.

30. C. E. Lewis and R. Easton, "Community medicine: Personality characteristics, career interests, observed health behavior, and teaching," *Arch. Environmental Health*, Vol. 21, July 1970, p. 99.

31. Richard. O. Rutland, "The family doctor's return," *Alabama Alumni News*, March, April 1962, p. 9.

32. Milford O. Rouse, M.D., "How to produce more doctors," *Today's Health*, May 1968: pp. 88–89.

33. Booz, Allen, Hamilton, Inc., "Expansion of Medical Education Programs in the State of Alabama. Special report," November 1967, p. 31.

34. John F. Burnum, "Early History and Founding of the College of Community Health Sciences," unpublished manuscript, date unknown.

35. Wolfe, p. 222.

36. Paul Davis, "Model hospital planned," *Tuscaloosa News*, March 11, 1970, p. 2.

37. Richard O. Rutland, speech delivered to Department of Behavioral and Community Medicine and RAHA, April 6, 1995.

38. See W. W. Winternitz and A. R. Gibbons, "Willard widened doctors' worlds," *Tuscaloosa News*, December 22, 1991, and W. W. Winternitz, A. R. Gibbons, and M. M. Hill, "Pioneer of Primary Care: William Willard, M.D.," *Yale Medicine*, Spring 1994, pp. 18–19.

39. See Robert Strauss, *A Medical School is Born* (Lexington: The University of Kentucky College of Medicine, 1996) for a thorough review of Willard's career at the University of Kentucky.

40. Speech by Julius B. Richmond, given at Willard's retirement, CCHS, Tuscaloosa, October 25, 1979.

41. W. R. Willard, commencement speech, date unknown.

42. Willard report, p.5.

43. W. R. Willard, "The Birth and Infancy of the College of Community Health Sciences," unpublished internal memorandum, p.16.

44. Rogers, Ward, Atkins, and Flynt, p. 580–81.

45. Willard, "Birth and Infancy," p. 18.

46. Ibid., p. 19.

47. Ibid., p. 49.

48. Ibid.

49. *Tuscaloosa News*, August 11, 1975, p. 1.

50. James A. Pittman, Jr., "The Dean's Report, University of Alabama School of Medicine, Spring 1975." *Alabama Journal of Medical Sciences*, Vol. 12, No. 2, 1975, p. 139.

51. Pittman, "Research and Health Care Reform," *The American Journal of the Medical Sciences*, May 1995, Vol. 309, Number 5, pp. 249–51.

52. Stephens, p. 22.

53. Ludmerer, *Time to Heal*, p. 135.

54. Willard, "Birth and Infancy," p. 129.

55. Ibid., p. 130.

56. Ibid.

57. Ibid., p. 132.

58. Brad Fisher, "Dean switched fish for school," *Tuscaloosa News*, September 2, 1979, p. 1, 3A.

59. Editorial, *Tuscaloosa News*, July 20, 1979, p. 4.

60. Riley Lumpkin, Letter to the editor, *Tuscaloosa News*, August 15, 1979, p. 4.

61. Anita Smith, "UA med school risks losing millions unless problems at Tuscaloosa corrected," *Birmingham News*, Oct. 17, 1979, p. 1.

62. Memorandum from D. T. McCall to Hill, Mathews, Wright, September 7, 1979.

63. Internal document, draft, "Comments on the Proposed Revision of the McCall Report Prepared by the CCHS Staff." September 14, 1979. It is not clear if anything came from this document or if it was even sent to the Board.

64. Letter to D. Mathews, S. Richardson Hill, and J. C. Wright from Joseph Volker, February 27, 1980.

65. College administrators decided that the name "Capstone Medical Center" more accurately described the many functions of the clinic, a medical group that offered internal medicine, pediatrics, obstetrics/gynecology, and family medicine.

66. For an excellent discussion on the creation of faculty practice plans, see Kenneth M. Ludmerer, *Time to Heal*, chapter 11.

67. Harry J. Knopke, Robert S. Northrup, and Julia A. Hartman, "BioPrep: A Premedical Program for Rural High School Students," *JAMA: Journal of the American Medical Association*, November 14, 1986, Vol. 256, p. 2549.

68. Letter from James A. Pittman, Jr., to James R. Schofield, Secretary, LCME. August 5, 1982. Progress report on the UA School of Medicine.

69. Rhonda Wooldridge, "Wallace opposes medical school student cutback," *Tuscaloosa News*, March 15, 1984, p. 1.

70. See William R. Willard, Elizabeth Ruben, and Harry J. Knopke, "Current practice characteristics and distribution patterns of Alabama physicians," *Journal of the Medical Association of the State of Alabama*, May 1983; Willard, Ruben, Knopke, "Projecting Alabama's Future Supply of Physicians," *Journal of the Medical Association of the State of Alabama*, June 1983.

71. Wilmer J. Coggins and Colleen Beall, "Medical Manpower in Alabama: Shortage, Sufficiency or Surfeit?," *Alabama Medicine, The Journal of MASA,* February 1989, p. 16.

72. Ibid.

73. See Barbara P. Doughty and Lisa R. Russell, "An AIDS Information Center," *Medical Reference Service Quarterly,* Vol. 8 (1), Spring 1989.

74. Willard, "Birth and Infancy," p. 23.

75. Linda Jackson, "OSCE uses standardized patients to test clinical skills," *On Rounds,* Vol. 6, no. 2, Fall 1996, p. 6.

76. Roland Ficken, Memo to Andrew Sorensen and Harold Fallon, June 25, 1996, p. 3.

77. Roland Ficken, "Dean's message," *On Rounds,* Vol. 2, no. 1, Winter 1992, p. 2.

78. Ficken, Memo to Sorensen and Fallon, p. 3

79. Richard Powell, "DCH likely to hold fast on funds it gives to UA," *Tuscaloosa News,* June 28, 1995, p. 1.

80. Roland Ficken, "Med school issue affects us all," *Tuscaloosa News,* July 23, 1995.

81. John Brandon and Garry Magouirk, memo to Bryan Kindred, DCH, June 14, 1995.

82. Linda Jackson, "Dean Ficken takes early retirement," *On Rounds,* Vol. 6, no. 1, Spring 1996, p. 1.

83. Ibid., p. 6.

84. Linda Jackson, "Curry named chair of internal medicine and UASOM assistant dean for rural medicine," *On Rounds,* Vol. 7, no. 2, Spring 1997, p. 2.

85. Linda Jackson, "Curry's delayed career in medical education benefits CCHS," *On Rounds,* Vol. 7, no. 3, Summer 1997, p. 7.

86. Linda Jackson, "New technology puts CCHS students and doctors at forefront of medical practice management," *On Rounds,* Vol. 12, no. 1, Winter 2002, p. 1.

87. Nabeel Memon and Brooke Taylor, "The medical school goes paperless: Enhancing access to information for improved patient care," *Joshua Journal of Science and Health* at the University of Alabama, Vol. 1, November 2002, p. 32.

88. Shannon Thomason, "UA hosts rural conference," *Tuscaloosa News,* April 25, 2000, p. 5A.

89. *Alabama Alumni Magazine,* March 2003, Vol. 83, no. 2, p. 5.

90. William Curry, "State of the College" address, Tuscaloosa, March 17, 2003.

91. Sarah Brotherton, Frank A. Simmons, and Sylvia I. Etzel, "U.S. Graduate Medical Education, 2000–2001, *JAMA: Journal of the American Medical Association,* September 5, 2001, Vol. 286, no. 9.

92. William T. Mallom, Mandy Liu, Robert F. Jones, and Michael Whitcomb, *Mini-Med: The Role of Regional Campuses in U.S. Medical Education* (Washington, DC: Association of American Medical Colleges, 2003), p. 6.

References

Books

Clark, Willis G. *History of Education in Alabama: 1702–1889.* Washington: Government Printing Office, 1889.

Fisher, Virginia E. *Building on a Vision: A Fifty-year Retrospective of UAB's Academic Health Center.* Birmingham: The University of Alabama at Birmingham, 1995.

Flexner, Abraham. *Medical Education in the United States and Canada.* New York: The Carnegie Foundation, 1910.

Harvey, Ira W. *A History of Educational Finance in Alabama.* Auburn: The Truman Pierce Institute, 1989.

Holley, Howard, M.D. *A History of Medicine in Alabama.* University: The University of Alabama Press, 1982.

Horsman, Reginald. *Josiah Nott of Mobile.* Baton Rouge: Louisiana State University Press, 1987.

Lewis, Irving J., and Cecil G. Sheps, M.D. *The Sick Citadel: The American Academic Medical Center and the Public Interest.* Cambridge: Oelgeschlager, Gunn & Hain, Publishers, Inc., 1983.

Ludmerer, Kenneth. *Learning to Heal.* New York: Basic Books, Inc., 1985.

———. *Time to Heal: American Medical Education from the Turn of the Century to the Era of Managed Care.* Oxford: Oxford University Press, 1999.

Mallom, William T., Mandy Liu, Robert F. Jones, and Michael Whitcomb. *Mini-Med: The Role of Regional Campuses in U.S. Medical Education.* Washington, DC: Association of American Medical Colleges, 2003.

Rogers, William Warren, Robert David Ward, Leah Rawls Atkins, and Wayne Flynt. *Alabama: History of a Deep South State.* Tuscaloosa: The University of Alabama Press, 1994.

Stephens, G. Gayle. *The Intellectual Basis of Family Practice.* Tucson, AZ: Winter Publishing Co., 1982.

Strauss, Robert. *A Medical School is Born.* Lexington: The University of Kentucky College of Medicine, 1996.

Willard, William R., M.D. *Medical Education and Medical Care in Alabama: Some Inadequacies, Some Solutions.* Tuscaloosa: The College of Community Health Sciences, 1983.

Wolfe, Suzanne Rau. *The University of Alabama: A Pictorial History.* University: University of Alabama Press, 1983.

Journal Articles

Alsobrook, David E. "Mobile v. Birmingham: The Alabama Medical College Controversy, 1912–1920." *The Alabama Review* (January 1983): 37–56.

Blair, A. W. "Spider poisoning: Experimental study of the effects of the bite of the female *Latrodectus mactans* in man," *Archives of Internal Medicine* 54, no. 6 (December 1934): 831–43.

Brotherton, Sarah, Frank A. Simmons, and Sylvia I. Etzel, "U.S. Graduate Medical Education, 2000–2001, *JAMA,* 286, no. 9 (September 5, 2001): 1056–60.

Coggins, Wilmer J., M.D., and Colleen Beall, "Medical Manpower in Alabama: Shortage, Sufficiency or Surfeit?," *Alabama Medicine, The Journal of MASA* (February 1989): 15–20.

Deuschle, Kurt, and Frederick Eberson, "Community medicine comes of age," *J. Med. Educ* 43 (December 1968): 1229–36.

Dohety, Barbara, and Lisa R. Russell, "An AIDS Information Center," *Medical Reference Services Quarterly,* Vol. 8, no. 1 (Spring 1989): 1–11.

Hiatt, Mark D. "Around the continent in 180 days: The controversial journey of Abraham Flexner," *The Pharos* (Winter 1999): pp. 18–24.

Knopke, Harry, Robert S. Northrup, and Julia A. Hartman, "BioPrep: A Premedical Program for Rural High School Students," *JAMA: Journal of the American Medical Association* 256 (November 14, 1986): 2548–51.

Lewis, C. E., and R. Easton, "Community medicine: Personality characteristics, career interests, observed health behavior, and teaching," *Arch. Environmental Health* 21 (July 1970): 99–104.

Ludmerer, Kenneth M. "The Rise of the Teaching Hospital in America." *Journal of the History of Medicine* 38 (October 1983): pp. 389–414.

Memon, Nabeel, and Brooke Taylor, "The medical school goes paperless: Enhancing access to information for improved patient care," *Joshua Journal of Science and Health at the University of Alabama* 1 (November 2002): 30–33.

Pittman, James A., Jr., "The Dean's Report, University of Alabama School of Medicine, Spring 1975." *Alabama Journal of Medical Sciences* 12, No. 2 (1975): 119–160.

———. "Research and Health Care Reform," *The American Journal of the Medical Sciences* 309, No. 5 (May 1995): p. 249–251.

Willard, William R., Elizabeth Ruben, and Harry J. Knopke, "Current practice characteristics and distribution patterns of Alabama physicians," *Journal of the Medical Association of the State of Alabama* (May 1983): 22–27.

———. "Projecting Alabama's Future Supply of Physicians," *Journal of the Medical Association of the State of Alabama* (June 1983): 12–18.

Magazine and Newspaper Articles

Alabama Alumni Magazine 83, no. 2 (March 2003): p. 5.

Author unknown, "University medical school dates back to 1859," *Crimson White,* 1931.

Davis, Paul. "Model hospital planned," *Tuscaloosa News,* March 11, 1970, p. 2.

Ficken, Roland. "Med school issue affects us all," *Tuscaloosa News* (July 23, 1995): 9A-10.

Fisher, Brad. "Dean switched fish for school," *Tuscaloosa News,* September 2, 1979. 1, 3A.

Jackson, Linda. "Dean Ficken takes early retirement," *On Rounds* 6, no. 1 (Spring 1996): 1.

———. "Curry named chair of internal medicine and UASOM assistant dean for rural medicine," *On Rounds* 7, no. 2 (Spring 1997): 1.

———. "New technology puts CCHS students and doctors at forefront of medical practice management," *On Rounds* 12, No. 1 (Winter 2002): 1, 3.

Lumpkin, Riley, M.D. Letter to the editor, *Tuscaloosa News* (August 15, 1979): 9.

Powell, Richard. "DCH likely to hold fast on funds it gives to UA," *Tuscaloosa News* (9 June 28, 1995): 1, 3B.

Rouse, Milford, O., M.D. "How to produce more doctors," *Today's Health,* Vol. 46 (May 1968): 88.

Rutland, Richard O., M.D. "The family doctor's return," *Alabama Alumni News* (March, April 1962): 7–9.

Schrag, Peter. "New beat in the heart of Dixie," *Saturday Review* (March 20, 1971): 42–45, 57–59.

Smith, Anita. "UA med school risks losing millions unless problems at Tuscaloosa corrected," *Birmingham News* (Oct. 17, 1979): 1.

Speagle, Scott M. "By process of elimination: The political decisions behind locating a four-year medical school in Birmingham." *The Vulcan Historical Review* 2 (Spring 1998): 48–70.

Thomason, Shannon. "UA hosts rural conference," *Tuscaloosa News* (April 25, 2000): 5A.

Winternitz, W. W., and A. R. Gibbons, "Willard widened doctors' worlds," *Tuscaloosa News,* December 22, 1991.

Winternitz, W. W., A. R. Gibbons and M. M. Hill, "Pioneer of primary care: William R. Willard, M.D." *Yale Medicine* (Spring 1994): 18–19.

Wooldridge, Rhonda. "Wallace opposes medical school student cutback," *Tuscaloosa News* (March 15, 1984): 1.

Memoirs, Speeches, and Miscellaneous Writings

Burnum, John F. "Early History and Founding of the College of Community Health Sciences," unpublished manuscript, date unknown.

Curry, William. "State of the College 2003," Speech delivered to faculty and staff of CCHS, March 19, 2003, Tuscaloosa, Alabama.

Graves, Stuart. Speech delivered to annual banquet of unnamed group, April 22, 1936, Montgomery, Alabama.

Richmond, Julius B. "Some thoughts on a quiet pioneer." Speech delivered in honor of William R. Willard, October 25, 1979. University of Alabama, Tuscaloosa, Alabama.

Rutland, Richard O. Speech delivered to Department of Behavioral and Community Medicine and RAHA, April 6, 1995. Tuscaloosa, Alabama.

Willard, William R. "The Birth and Infancy of the College of Community Health Sciences." Unpublished manuscript, undated.

Manuscript Collections

University of Alabama Library

David Mathews papers
Frank A. Rose papers
Roger Sayers papers
Joab Thomas papers
College of Community Health Sciences files

University of Alabama at Birmingham Library

James A. Pittman papers

Personal Papers

T. Riley Lumpkin, M.D.
John Packard, M.D.

Reports

Ad Hoc Committee on Education for Family Practice. 1966. "Meeting the Challenge of Family Practice" [known as "the Willard report"]. Chicago: Council of Medical Education, American Medical Association.

Booz, Allen, and Hamilton, Inc. 1967. "Expansion of Medical Education Programs in the State of Alabama." A special report prepared at the request of the Alabama Legislature. November.

Coggeshall, Lewis T., M.D. "Planning for Medical Progress through Education." 1965. Report submitted to Executive Council of the Association of American Medical Colleges. Evanston, IL. April.

The Graduate Education of Physicians. 1966. "The Report of the Citizens Commission on Graduate Medical Education." Chicago: American Medical Association.

Interviews

		Interviewer
Chelley Alexander, M.D.,	Faculty, Family Medicine Assistant Residency Director	Coggins
Russell Anderson, M.D.,	Former Chair, Family Medicine Former Associate Dean for Academic Affairs	Coggins

Marc Armstrong, M.D.*	Faculty, Family Medicine Medical Director, CMC	Coggins
John Brandon, M.D.*	Private practice, Family Medicine, Adjunct Associate Professor CCHS	Coggins
Alan Blum, M.D.	Professor, and Gerald Leon Wallace Endowed Chair in Family Medicine	Coggins
Elizabeth Cockrum, M.D.*	Associate Professor, Pediatrics	Coggins
Robert Centor, M.D.	Former Dean, CCHS, Professor of Internal Medicine, UASOM	Coggins
Shirley Culp	Former Administrative Assistant, CCHS	Ficken
William Curry, M.D.	Dean and Chair of Internal Medicine	Coggins
William Deal, M.D.	Dean, UASOM	Coggins
Daveta Dozier, M.D.*	Private Practice Thomasville, AL	Coggins
Frank Dozier, M.D.*	Private Practice Thomasville, AL	Coggins
Shirley Florence	Former Administrative Assistant to the Dean of CCHS	Coggins
Harold Fallon, M.D.	Dean Emeritus, UASOM	Ficken
James Ford	Former Chief Executive Officer, DCH	Coggins
Margaret Garner	M.S., R.D., CCHS Director of Nutrition Education and Services Family Medicine	Coggins

*Indicates former student and/or resident at CCHS.

David Hefelfinger, M.D.	Former Chair, Pediatrics Former Associate Dean for Clinical Affairs	Coggins
John Higginbotham, Ph.D.	Interim Chair, Community and Rural Medicine	Coggins
Dwight Hooper, M.D.	Chair, OB/GYN	Coggins
Robert Ireland, M.D.*	Associate Professor, Family Medicine	Coggins
Diane Kerr, L.P.N.	Team Leader, CMC	Coggins
James Leeper, Ph.D.	Former Chair, Community & Rural Medicine, Professor	Coggins
T. Riley Lumpkin, M.D.	Professor Emeritus, Family Medicine Former Associate Dean, Continuing Medical Education	Coggins
E. Eugene Marsh, M.D.	Associate Dean for Academic Affairs	Coggins
David Mathews, Ph.D.	President Emeritus, UA	Ficken
John Maxwell, B.A.	Administrator, CMC	Coggins
Jerry McKnight, M.D.*	Former Chair, Family Medicine Associate Professor	Coggins
Robert Moore, Ph.D.	Former Assistant Dean for Administrative Affairs	Coggins
W. Larry Rainey, Ph.D.	Former Assistant Director, Director, BioPrep Program	Coggins
Laura Satcher, M.D.*	Assistant Professor, Family Medicine	Coggins
Roger Sayers, Ph.D.	President Emeritus, UA	Ficken
C. William Scott, Jr., M.D.	UASOM	Coggins/ Ficken

Mary Leta Taylor	Former Administrative Assistant, Medical Student Affairs	Coggins
Michael Taylor, M.D.	Chair, Dept. of Pediatrics	Coggins
Joab Thomas, Ph.D.	President Emeritus, UA	Coggins
Carolyn Watson, B.A.	Former Administrative Assistant to the Dean	Coggins
John R. Wheat, M.D., M.P.H.	Professor, Community and Rural Medicine	Coggins

Index

Page numbers in boldface refer to illustrations.